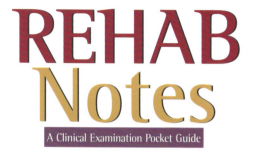

REHAB
Notes
A Clinical Examination Pocket Guide

Ellen Hillegass, PT, PhD

Purchase additional copies of this book at your health science bookstore or directly from F. A. Davis by shopping online at www.fadavis.com or by calling 800-323-3555 (US) or 800-665-1148 (CAN)

A Davis's Notes Book

F. A. Davis Company
1915 Arch Street
Philadelphia, PA 19103
www.fadavis.com

Printed in China by Imago

Last digit indicates print number: 10 9 8 7 6 5 4 3 2

Acquisitions Editor: Margaret Biblis
Developmental Editors: Melissa Reed and Maria Sussman
Manager of Art & Design: Carolyn O'Brien
Reviewers: Frank B. Underwood, PT, PhD, ECS; Kristen Geissler, MS, PT, CPHQ;
Edmund M. Kosmahl, PT, EdD; Steven Raymond Tippet, PhD, PT, SCS, ATC;
Jennifer Ellison, PhD, PT, Reed Humphrey, PhD, PT, Cindy Flom-Meland, PT, PhD,
NCS; Ronald De Vera Barredo, PT, EdD, DPT, GCS; Gordon Alderink, PT, PhD.

As new scientific information becomes available through basic and clinical
research, recommended treatments and drug therapies undergo changes. The
author(s) and publisher have done everything possible to make this book accurate,
up to date, and in accord with accepted standards at the time of publication. The
author(s), editors, and publisher are not responsible for errors or omissions or for
consequences from application of the book, and make no warranty, expressed or
implied, in regard to the contents of the book. Any practice described in this book
should be applied by the reader in accordance with professional standards of care
used in regard to the unique circumstances that may apply in each situation. The
reader is advised always to check product information (package inserts) for
changes and new information regarding dose and contraindications before
administering any drug. Caution is especially urged when using new or
infrequently ordered drugs.

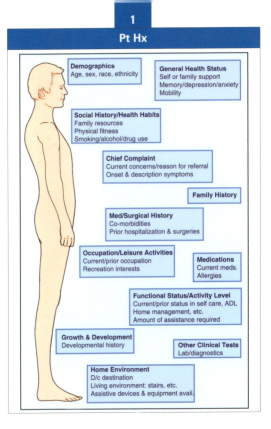

1

Pt Hx

Demographics
Age, sex, race, ethnicity

General Health Status
Self or family support
Memory/depression/anxiety
Mobility

Social History/Health Habits
Family resources
Physical fitness
Smoking/alcohol/drug use

Chief Complaint
Current concerns/reason for referral
Onset & description symptoms

Family History

Med/Surgical History
Co-morbidities
Prior hospitalization & surgeries

Occupation/Leisure Activities
Current/prior occupation
Recreation interests

Medications
Current meds.
Allergies

Functional Status/Activity Level
Current/prior status in self care, ADL
Home management, etc.
Amount of assistance required

Growth & Development
Developmental history

Other Clinical Tests
Lab/diagnostics

Home Environment
D/c destination
Living environment: stairs, etc.
Assistive devices & equipment avail.

Chief Complaint & Symptom Hx

- Description of onset of symptoms
- Duration of symptoms
- Factors that increase symptoms
- Factors that decrease symptoms
- Associated symptoms

General Demographics

- Age:
- Sex:
  - Male
  - Female
- Race:
  - White
  - African American
  - Hispanic
  - Asian
  - Other
- Primary language:
  - English
  - Spanish
  - French
  - German
  - Japanese
  - Chinese
  - Other
- Education level:
  - K-12; completed grade
  - Undergraduate education
  - Graduate education

Social/Environment Hx

- Family/caregiver resources
- Social supports
- Living environment:
    - Single home
    - Apartment/condominium
    - Senior independent living
    - Assisted living
    - Nursing home
    - Other
- Discharge destination:
    - Same
    - Other
- Social habits:
    - Drinks alcohol   Yes   No if yes # drinks/wk _____
    - Smokes cigarettes   Yes   No if yes # cigarettes/day _____
    - If no, former smoker?   Yes   No
    - If yes: # ppd # yr smoked _____
    - Illegal drug use _____
- Physical fitness: Exercises regularly   Yes   No

Employment/Occupation

- Currently employed: Yes   No
- Full-time/part-time/other _____
- Occupation: _____
- Retired: Yes   No
- If retired, former occupation: _____
- Leisure activities: list

_____

_____

_____

_____

_____

Past Medical Hx, Including Surgeries, etc.

- Previous hospitalizations
- Previous surgeries
- Previous medical problems
- Past medical status of problems with:

- Cardiovascular
- Endocrine/metabolic
- Gastrointestinal
- Genitourinary
- Gynecological
- Integumentary

- Musculoskeletal
- Neuromuscular
- Obstetric
- Psychological
- Pulmonary

Fam Medical Hx

- Fam hx of cardiovascular disease (angina, heart attack, stroke, heart failure, PVD)
  - Age of first Dx _____
- Fam hx of diabetes
- Fam hx of cancer? What type of cancer? _____
  Other fam hx _____

Functional Status

- Current & prior status in self-care & home management (ADL)
  - Work
- Independent
- Requires assistance for self-care or home management
- Dependent in care

Medication

- Medications for current condition
- Medication for other condition

4

Assessment of Risk Factors: Falling, Cardiac Disease, Pulmonary Disease, DVT, & Skin Problems

Risk Factors for Falling

Age Changes	Medications

Muscle weakness
Decreased balance
Impaired proprioception
  or sensation
Delayed muscle response
  time/increased reaction
  time
	Antihypertensives
	Sedative-hypnotics
	Antidepressants
	Antipsychotics
	Diuretics
	Narcotics
	Use of more than four medications

Environmental	**Pathological Conditions**

Poor lighting
Throw rugs, loose carpet,
  complex carpet designs
Cluster of wires/cords
Stairs w/o handrails
Bathrooms w/o grab rails
Slippery floors
Restraints
Footwear (slippers)
Use of alcohol
	Vestibular disorders
	Orthostatic hypotension (especially
	  before breakfast)
	Neuropathies
	Osteoarthritis
	Osteoporosis
	Visual or hearing impairment
	Cardiovascular disease
	Urinary incontinence
	CNS disorders (stroke, Parkinson's
	  disease, multiple sclerosis)

Other	
Elder abuse/assault Nonambulatory status Gait changes (decreased stride length or speed) Postural instability Fear of falling	

Risk Factors for Heart Disease

Risk Factors for CAD	Major = ** Minor = *	Absence = − Fam Hx = Fam	Presence = +
Hypertension >140 systolic or >90 diastolic	**		
Smoking (# ppd × # yr)	**		
Elevated cholesterol Total >200, LDL >160 & no CAD or LDL >100 w/CAD HDL <40 males, HDL <50 females	**		
Sedentary lifestyle	**		
Fam hx (1 or more parent <60 yr when dx w/CAD, MI, stroke)	**		
Diabetes	**		
Stress (anger/hostility)	*		
Age (older)	*		
Obesity or elevated BMI	*		
Sex (M or menopausal F)	*		
Elevated triglycerides >150	*		

Risk Factors for Pulmonary Disease

Risk Factors for Pulmonary Disease	Presence (+)/Absence(−)
Smoking (ppd × yr smoked)	
Occupational/environmental exposure	
Toxic fumes: chlorine, chemicals, formaldehyde, plant nursery chemicals, etc.	
Dusts: carpentry work, asbestos, coal, silica	
Family hx of asthma	
Alpha-$_1$ antitrypsin deficiency	
AIDS/ARDS	

Risk Factors for Skin Breakdown

- Amputation
- Congestive heart failure
- Diabetes
- Malnutrition
- Neuromuscular dysfunction
- Obesity
- Peripheral nerve involvement
- Polyneuropathy
- Prior scar
- Spinal cord involvement
- Surgery
- Vascular
- Altered mentation/coma
- Decreased level of activity
- Decreased sensation
- Edema
- Inflammation
- Ischemia
- Pain

Symptoms of DVT	Symptoms of Pulmonary Embolism
Swelling of leg	Shortness of breath
Warmth & redness of leg	Chest pain, w/deep breaths
Pain, noticeable when standing/walking	Coughing up phlegm w/blood; streaking/flecks

ASSESS & EVAL

Risk Factors for DVT

DVT more likely to occur in people:

- Age >40 yr
- Prolonged bed rest (immobility)
- Major injuries or paralysis
- Surgery, especially leg joints or pelvis
- Cancer & its treatments
- Long-distance travel: prolonged immobility
- Pregnancy/childbirth: due to hormone changes; risk highest just after childbirth
- Using contraceptives w/estrogen
- HRT
- Other circulation or heart problems

Direction of flow

Vein wall

Build-up of thrombus

Deep vein thrombosis

Systems Review

Cardiovascular/Pulmonary	NL	ABN
Resting BP (<140/90)		
Resting HR (<100 beats/min)		
Resting RR (<16 breaths/min)		
Edema ■ Bilateral ■ Unilateral		
Integumentary		
Pliability (texture)		
Presence of scar formation		
Skin color		
Skin integrity		
Musculoskeletal NL ROM & Strength		
Gross ROM UE		
LE		
Gross strength UE		
LE		
Symmetry		
Height		
Wt		
BMI		

(Continued text on following page)

Systems Review (Continued)

Neuromuscular	NL	ABN
Gross coordinated movements		
Balance		
Sitting ■		
Standing ■		
Gait		
Locomotion		
Transfers		
Transitions		
Motor function/motor control		
Gastrointestinal/Genitourinary		
■ Heartburn, diarrhea, vomiting, abdominal pain		
■ Menstrual problems, pregnancy		
■ Swallowing problems		
■ Bladder problems		
Communication/Affect/Cognition/Language/Learning Style		
Ability to make needs known		
Consciousness		
Expected emotional/behavioral responses		
Learning preferences/education needs/barriers		
Orientation (person, place, time)		
General		
Unexplained wt loss or gain		
Fever, chills, fatigue		

Tests & Measures: Areas in Systems Review Requiring Further Assessment (see specific tabs)

Cardiovascular & Pulmonary

- ■ Aerobic capacity/endurance tests
  - ■ Functional capacity during ADLs
    - • Standardized exercise testing protocols
      - – 6-minute walk test
- ■ Cardiovascular signs & symptoms in response to increased O_2 demand w/exercise or activity
  - ■ HR, rhythm, heart sounds
  - ■ BP, arterial pressures, blood flow (w/Doppler)
  - ■ Perceived exertion w/activities
  - ■ Angina, claudication assessments
- ■ Pulmonary signs & symptoms in response to increased O_2 demand w/activity or exercise
  - ■ Dyspnea   ■ SpO_2
  - ■ Ventilatory pattern ■ Cyanosis, gas exchange, gas analysis
- ■ Physiological responses to position change, including autonomic responses, central, & peripheral pressures
- ■ Pulmonary signs of ventilatory function
  - ■ Airway protection
  - ■ Breath & voice sounds
  - ■ Respiratory rate, rhythm, & pattern
  - ■ Ventilatory flow, forces, & volumes
  - ■ Airway clearance assessment

Neuromuscular

- ■ Cranial & peripheral nerve integrity
- ■ Dynamometry
- ■ Specific muscle tests
- ■ Thoracic outlet tests

(Continued text on following page)

Neuromuscular (Continued)

- Response to neural provocation
- Tension tests
- Vertebral artery compression
- Response to stimuli (auditory, gustatory, olfactory, pharyngeal, vestibular, & visual)
- Sensory distribution of cranial & peripheral nerves
- Discrimination tests
- Tactile tests
  - Coarse vs. light touch
  - Cold vs. heat tests
  - Pressure/vibration tests
- Dexterity, coordination, & agility tests
- Electroneuromyography
- Hand function: fine vs. gross motor, finger dexterity
- Initiation, modification, & control of movement patterns
- Developmental scales
  - Movement assessment batteries
  - Postural challenge tests
- Musculoskeletal
  - Joint integrity & mobility
  - Apprehension, compression, & distraction
  - Drawer, glide, impingement, shear, & valgus/varus stress tests
  - Joint play movements
  - Muscle strength, power, & endurance tests
  - Muscle tension (palpation)
  - Muscle length, soft tissue extensibility, & flexibility tests
- Posture evaluation
- Integumentary
  - Activities, positions, & postures that produce or relieve trauma
  - Assessment of devices/equipment that produce or relieve trauma to skin
  - Skin characteristics
    - Blistering
    - Mobility of skin
    - Dermatitis
    - Nail growth
    - Hair growth
    - Temperature, texture, turgor

Neuromuscular *(Continued)*

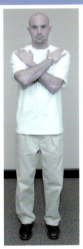

Standing balance test. Pt should maintain position w/o moving or swaying.

0 1 2 3 4 5 6 7 8 9 10

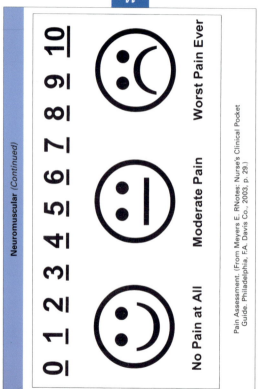

No Pain at All   Moderate Pain   Worst Pain Ever

Pain Assessment. (From Meyers E. RNotes: Nurse's Clinical Pocket
Guide. Philadelphia, F.A. Davis Co., 2003; p. 29.)

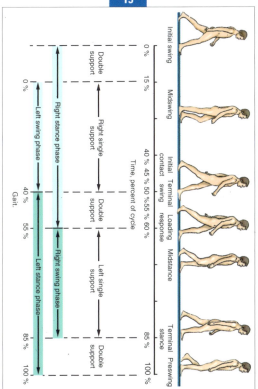

Gait.

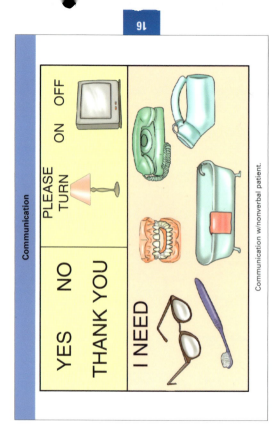

Communication

YES NO	PLEASE TURN	ON OFF
THANK YOU		
I NEED		

Communication w/nonverbal patient.

Functional Assessment & Impairment Terminology	
Definitions	
Independent	Pt able to consistently perform skill safely w/no one present & no cuing
Supervison	Pt requires one person w/in arm's reach as precaution; ↓ probability of requiring assistance
Close guarding	Person positioned to assist w/hands raised but not touching pt; fair probability of requiring assistance
Minimum assist	Pt completes **majority** of activity w/o assist
Moderate assist	Pt completes **part** of activity w/o assist
Maximum assist	Pt unable to assist in any part of activity

Balance Definitions: Sitting or Standing	
NL	Maintains position w/maximal disturbance
Good	Maintains position w/moderate disturbance
Fair	Maintains position unsupported: short period
Poor	Attempts to assist: requires assist to maintain
None	Unable to assist in maintaining position

Functional Tests	Assistance		
Bed mobility	Rolling side to side		
	Scooting up & down in bed		
Transfers	Supine↔Sidelying↔Sit		
	Sit↔Stand		
	Stand pivot sit		
	Wheelchair↔toilet		
	Wheelchair↔tub		
Balance	Sitting		
	Standing		
	Dynamic		
Ambulation	w/Assistive device		
	w/o Assistive device		

Special Considerations w/All Populations: Alerts/Indicators

Effects of Bedrest

↑ VO$_2$ max	Muscle atrophy
↑ Plasma volume	↑ Muscle tone
↑ Red cell mass	↑ Muscle endurance
↑ Stroke volume	Bone demineralization
↑ Maximal exercise cardiac output	↑ Insulin sensitivity
↑ Oxidative capacity of muscle	↑ Carbohydrate tolerance
↑ Orthostatic tolerance	↓ Serum lipids
↑ Vasomotor function	Altered immune system function
↑ Heat tolerance	↓ Susceptibility to renal infection, DVT, sleep disturbance
↑ Nitrogen balance in skeletal muscle	

Effects of Aging
Effects on Body Functions

↓ Peak Vo₂ (aerobic capacity)	↓ 20%-30% by age 80 yr
↓ Cardiac index	↓ 20%-30% by age 80 yr
↓ Max breathing capacity	↓ 40%
↓ Liver & kidney function	↓ 40%-50%
↓ Bone mass	↓ 15% in men, 30% in women
↓ Muscle strength	↓ 20%-30%
↓ Joint flexibility	↓ 20%-30%
↓ Endocrine function	↓ 40%
↓ # Spinal cord axons	↓ 37%
↓ Nerve conduction velocity	↓ 10%-15%

Early Warning Cancer Signs (American Cancer Society)

- Changes in bowel or bladder habits
- A sore that does not heal in 6 wk
- Unusual bleeding or discharge
- Thickening or lump in breast or elsewhere
- Indigestion or difficulty in swallowing
- Obvious change in wart or mole
- Nagging cough or hoarseness
- Proximal muscle weakness
- Change in deep tendon reflexes

Other screening clues:

- Previous personal hx of any cancer
- Recent wt loss of 10 lb or more within 1 mo
- Constant pain, unrelieved by rest or change in position
- Night pain
- Development of new neurological deficits
- Changes in size, shape, tenderness, & consistency of lymph nodes, painless & present in >1 location
- Any woman w/chest, breast, axillary, or shoulder pain of unknown cause

Types of Cancer

Type	Etiology/Location
Adenocarcinoma	Glandular tissue
Carcinoma	Epithelial tissue
Glioma	Brain, supportive tissue, spinal cord
Leukemia	Blood-forming cells
Lymphoma	Lymphatic cells
Melanoma	Pigment cells
Myeloma	Plasma cells
Sarcoma	Mesenchymal cells

Cancer Staging (TNM)

T = tumor, N = node, M = metastasis

T1 = small, confined	N0 = no other involvement	M0 = no metastasis
T2–T3 = medium	N1–3 = moderate involvement	M1 = metastasis
T4 = large	N4 = extensive	

Diabetes Assessment

Characteristics	Type I	Type II
Onset	In childhood or young adulthood	Adult onset, >40 yr
Etiology	Little or no insulin production by beta cells of islets of Langerhans	Partial ↓ of insulin production or ↑ sensitivity of tissues to insulin
Treatment	Insulin-dependent	Noninsulin-dependent, may be controlled w/diet, exercise, & wt loss

Estimated New Cancer Cases
10 Leading Sites by Sex, United States, 2005

Prostate 33%	32% Breast
Lung and bronchus 13%	12% Lung and bronchus
Colon and rectum 10%	11% Colon and rectum
Urinary bladder 7%	6% Uterine carpus
Melanoma of skin 5%	4% Non-Hodgkin's lymphoma
Non-Hodgkin's lymphoma 4%	4% Melanoma of skin
Kidney and renal pelvis 3%	3% Ovary
Leukemia 3%	3% Thyroid
Oral cavity and pharynx 3%	2% Urinary bladder
Pancreas 2%	2% Pancreas
All other sites 17%	21% All other sites

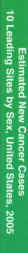

Estimated New Cancer Cases
10 Leading Sites by Sex, United States, 2005

Male			Female	
Lung and bronchus	31%		Lung and bronchus	27%
Prostate	10%		Breast	15%
Colon and rectum	10%		Colon and rectum	10%
Pancreas	5%		Ovary	6%
Leukemia	4%		Pancreas	6%
Esophagus	4%		Leukemia	4%
Liver and intrahepatic bile duct	3%		Non-Hodgkin's lymphoma	3%
Non-Hodgkin's lymphoma	3%		Uterine corpus	3%
Urinary bladder	3%		Multiple myeloma	2%
Kidney and renal pelvis	3%		Brain and other nervous system	2%
All other sites	24%		All other sites	22%

Signs/Symptoms of Hypoglycemia

Adrenergic Signs/Symptoms	Neuroglucopenic Signs/Symptoms
Weakness	Headache
Sweating	Hypothermia
Tachycardia	Visual disturbances
Palpitations	Mental dullness
Tremor	Confusion
Nervousness	Amnesia
Irritability	Seizures
Tingling mouth & fingers	Coma
Hunger	
Nausea	
Vomiting	

Signs of Physical Abuse

Signs & symptoms of physical abuse in the elderly:

- Bruises, black eyes, welts, lacerations, & rope marks
- Bone fractures, broken bones, & skull fractures
- Open wounds, cuts, punctures, untreated injuries in various stages of healing
- Sprains, dislocations, & internal injuries/bleeding
- Broken eyeglasses/frames, physical signs of being subjected to punishment, & signs of being restrained
- Laboratory findings of medication overdose or underutilization of prescribed drugs
- An elder's report of being hit, slapped, kicked, or mistreated
- An elder's sudden change in behavior
- The caregiver's refusal to allow visitors to see an elder alone

Some signs of physical abuse in children & adolescents:

- Unexplained burns, cuts, bruises, or welts in the shape of an object
- Bite marks
- Antisocial behavior
- Problems in school
- Fear of adults
- Drug or alcohol abuse
- Self-destructive or suicidal behavior
- Depression or poor self-image

Some signs of emotional abuse:

- Apathy
- Depression
- Hostility
- Lack of concentration
- Eating disorders
- Inappropriate interest in or knowledge of sexual acts
- Seductiveness
- Avoidance of things related to sexuality or rejection of own genitals or body
- Nightmares & bedwetting
- Drastic changes in appetite
- Overcompliance or excessive aggression
- Fear of a particular person or fam member
- Withdrawal, secretiveness, or depression
- Suicidal behavior
- Eating disorders
- Self-injury
- Substance abuse
- Running away
- Inhibited behavior
- Disturbed play
- Aggression

Nutritional Needs Assesment

% Ideal Body Wt. _____ BMI _____
Wt. change: Mild _____ Moderate _____
Severe _____
Available lab reports: Albumin _____ Cholesterol:
_____ Glucose: _____
Possible drug/nutrient reactions? _____

Comments/Assessment _____

Nutritional Needs Assessment *(Continued)*

Indicators of Nutritional Problems

	Yes	No
Significant wt change ($+/-$ 10 lb or $>$ in past year)		
Intermittent or continuous use of steroids		
>30% BMI		
Changes in eating habits recently		
Follows dietary restrictions		
Food allergies		
Problems with: Dental		
Chewing		
Swallowing		
Digestion		
Constipation/diarrhea		
Inadequate intake of fluids (<8 cups or 64 oz/day)		
Low albumin/prealbumin		

Red flags for potential feeding difficulties:
- Slow feeding progression
- Respiratory difficulties
- Spits out food
- Oral touch sensitive
- Coughs frequently
- Hypersensitive gag
- Tube feeding beyond 2 mo
- Persistent reflexes
- Jaw moves excessively
- ABN muscle tone
- Color change w/feeding
- Poor transition to solids

Red flags for swallowing difficulties:
- Hx of respiratory difficulties
- Pneumonias
- Muscle tone abnormalities
- Anoxic events
- Traumatic brain injury
- Ventilator dependence
- Apnea
- Stridor
- Color changes
- Coughing during or after feeding
- Poor handling of secretions
- Slow growth pattern

Body Mass Index Table

	Normal						Overweight					Obese										Extreme obesity		
BMI	19	20	21	22	23	24	25	26	27	28	29	30	31	32	33	34	35	36	37	38	39	40	41	42
Height (inches)												Body Weight (pounds)												
58	91	96	100	105	110	115	119	124	129	134	138	143	148	153	158	162	167	172	177	181	186	191	196	201
59	94	99	104	109	114	119	124	128	133	138	143	148	153	158	163	168	173	178	183	188	193	198	203	208
60	97	102	107	112	118	123	128	133	138	143	148	153	158	163	168	174	179	184	189	194	199	204	209	215
61	100	106	111	116	122	127	132	137	143	148	153	158	164	169	174	180	185	190	195	201	206	211	217	222
62	104	109	115	120	126	131	136	142	147	153	158	164	169	175	180	186	191	196	202	207	213	218	224	229
63	107	113	118	124	130	135	141	146	152	158	163	169	175	180	186	191	197	203	208	214	220	225	231	237
64	110	116	122	128	134	140	145	151	157	163	169	174	180	186	192	197	204	209	215	221	227	232	238	244
65	114	120	126	132	138	144	150	156	162	168	174	180	186	192	198	204	210	216	222	228	234	240	246	252
66	118	124	130	136	142	148	155	161	167	173	179	186	192	198	204	210	216	223	229	235	241	247	253	260
67	121	127	134	140	146	153	159	166	172	178	185	191	198	204	211	217	223	230	236	242	249	255	261	268
68	125	131	138	144	151	158	164	171	177	184	190	197	203	210	216	223	230	236	243	249	256	262	269	276
69	128	135	142	149	155	162	169	176	182	189	196	203	209	216	223	230	236	243	250	257	263	270	277	284
70	132	139	146	153	160	167	174	181	188	195	202	209	216	222	229	236	243	250	257	264	271	278	285	292
71	136	143	150	157	165	172	179	186	193	200	208	215	222	229	236	243	250	257	265	272	279	286	293	301
72	140	147	154	162	169	177	184	191	199	206	213	221	228	235	242	250	258	265	272	279	287	294	302	309
73	144	151	159	166	174	182	189	197	204	212	219	227	235	242	250	257	265	272	280	288	295	302	310	318
74	148	155	163	171	179	186	194	202	210	218	225	233	241	249	256	264	272	280	287	295	303	311	319	326
75	152	160	168	176	184	192	200	208	216	224	232	240	248	256	264	272	279	287	295	303	311	319	327	335
76	156	164	172	180	189	197	205	213	221	230	238	246	254	263	271	279	287	295	304	312	320	328	336	344

BMI = body mass (kg)/height (m)

Assessment of BMI. (Adapted from Clinical Guidelines on the Identification, Evaluation, and Treatment of Overweight and Obesity in Adults: The Evidence Report. NIH publication 98-4083, September 1998.)

Pt Education Needs Assessment Checklist

- Understanding of disease
- Knowledge of medications: indications & side effects
- Activity limitations
- Signs/symptoms to anticipate
- Action to take w/signs/symptoms
- Knowledge of when to call doctor/ER

Additional Pt Resources

- Dietitian
- Case Mgr/social worker
- Psychologist/behav specialist
- Other specialist

Hospital/Home
Adaptive Equipment Chart

Equipment	Have	Need	Special Considerations
Hospital bed			
Wheelchair ■ Manual/electric			
Mobility ■ Cane: straight			
4-pronged ■ Walker: pickup ■ 2 wheels			
■ 4 wheels			
Raised toilet seat			
Shower chair			
Shower/bath stool			
Electric bed			
Grab bars in bathroom			
Other			

Adaptive Equipment & Environment Dimensions

Wheelchair dimensions	
■ Overall height	36-37 in
■ Seat depth	16-17 in
■ Footrest support	16-22 in
■ Armrest height	5-12 in
■ Seat height from floor	19.5-20.5 in
■ Seat & back width	14-22 in
Wheelchair clearance for door	36 in min
Turning space for wheelchair	60-78 in min
Closet: hanging or shelf heights	48 in max
Drinking fountains spout height	36 in max
Bathroom stall	60 × 96 in
Bathtubs: clear space out of tub	60 × 30 in

Procedural Interventions

■ ADL training
■ Aerobic capacity/endurance conditioning or reconditioning
■ Airway clearance techniques
■ Balance, coordination, & agility training
■ Body mechanics & postural stabilization
■ Breathing strategies
■ Coordination, communication, & documentation
■ Devices & equipment use & training
■ Electrotherapeutic modalities
■ Flexibility exercise
■ Functional training programs in self-care, home management,
  work community, & leisure
■ Gait & locomotion training
■ Injury prevention or reduction
■ Integumentary repair & protection techniques
■ Manual therapy techniques & mobilization/manipulation
■ Neuromotor development training
■ Pt-/client-related instruction

- Physical agents & mechanical modalities
- Positioning
- Prescription, application & fabrication of devices & equipment
- Relaxation training
- Strength, power, & endurance training for skeletal & ventilatory muscles

APTA: Guide to Physical Therapist Practice, 2nd ed., Physical Therapy 2001;81;9-744.

Anticipated or Expected Outcomes

- Ability to perform physical actions/tasks/activities improved
- Ability to perform, assume or resume required self-care, home management, work, etc., improved
- Aerobic capacity improved
- Airway clearance improved
- Atelectasis ↓
- Balance improved
- Cough improved
- Edema, lymphedema, or effusion ↓
- Endurance increased
- Energy expenditure per unit of work ↓
- Exercise tolerance improved
- Fitness improved
- Gait, locomotion, & balance improved
- Health status improved
- Integumentary integrity improved
- Joint integrity & mobility improved
- Joint swelling, inflammation, or restriction reduced
- Level of supervision required for task performance ↓
- Motor function (motor control & motor learning) improved
- Muscle performance (strength, power, & endurance) ↑
- Optimal joint alignment achieved
- Optimal loading on a body part achieved
- Pain decreased
- Performance of ADLs with or w/o assistive devices ↑
- Physical function improved

ASSESS & EVAL

- Physiological response to ↑ O_2 demand improved
- Postural control improved
- Pre- & postoperative complications ↓
- Quality & quantity of movement of body segments improved
- ROM improved
- Relaxation ↑
- Risk of secondary impairment ↓
- Risk factors for disease ↓
- Self-management of symptoms improved
- Sensory awareness ↑
- Soft tissue swelling, inflammation, or restriction ↓
- Tissue perfusion & oxygenation enhanced
- Tolerance of positions & activities ↑
- Use of physical therapy services optimized
- Use & cost of health care services ↓
- Weight-bearing status improved
- Work of breathing ↓

APTA: Guide to Physical Therapist Practice, 2nd ed. Physical Therapy 2001:81;9-744.

Discharge: Expected

**Assessment of Planned Destination:
Acute Rehab/Skilled Care/Home**

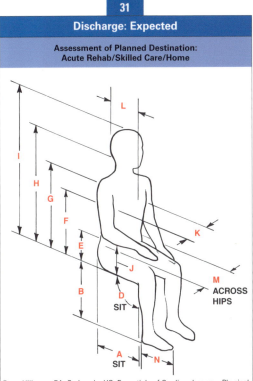

From Hillegass EA, Sadowsky HS. Essentials of Cardiopulmonary Physical
Therapy, 2/e. WB Saunders, Philadelphia, 2001.

Auscultation	
Breath Sounds	**Interpretation**
Adequate sound, pitch, intensity on inspir & expir: no ABN sounds	NL
↓ sounds	Hyperinflated lungs: COPD Hypoinflation: acute lung disease (e.g., atelectasis, pneumothorax, pleural effusion)
Absent sounds	Pleural effusion, pneumothorax, obesity, 3rd trimester pregnancy in lower lobes, **severe** hyperinflation as in COPD
Bronchial breath sounds	Consolidation (pneumonia), large atelectasis w/patent airway adjacent
Wheezes (rhonchi)	Diffuse airway obstruction usually associated w/bronchospasm or tumor OR localized stenosis
Crackles (rales)	Secretions present if on inspiration & expiration; atelectasis if on inspiration only
↓ voice sounds (repeating 99 or A)	Atelectasis, pleural effusion, pneumothorax
↑ voice sounds	Consolidation, pulmonary fibrosis
Extrapulmonary adventitious sound: pleural rub	Pleural inflammation or pleuritis

Assessment of Phonation, Cough, & Sputum

Assessments	ABN Findings & Interpretation
Phonation	Dyspnea of phonation Count words expressed before next breath Poor voice control: weak musculature
Cough	Ineffective: assess for weakness of musculature & pain Productive of secretions: evaluate secretions & chronicity of secretions Violent/spasmatic: may be aspiration or bronchospasm Nonproductive but persistent: auscultate: assess for signs of infection, pulm fibrosis, pulm infiltrates
Sputum	Evaluate color: white/clear: noninfected Blood-tinged: could be irritation of trachea/bronchi, TB, fungal Frank blood: neoplastic or pulmonary infarct Evaluate consistency: Copious: long-standing problem Thick, formerly mucoid: acute/exacerbation, may be dehydrated as well Frothy: pulm edema/heart failure Evaluate smell: bronchiectasis/infective Evaluate amt: ↑ from NL indicates acute exacerbation
Breath	Foul-smelling: anaerobic infection of mouth/respiratory tract Acetone: ketoacidosis

Cardiopulmonary Assessment

Evaluation of Breathing

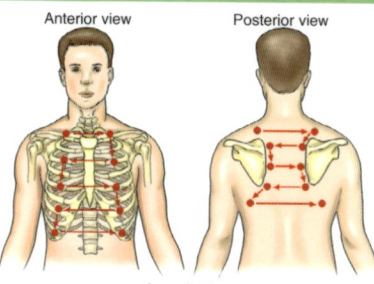

Anterior view   Posterior view

Auscultation.

Errors of auscultation to avoid:
- Listening to breath sounds through pt gown
- Allowing tubing to rub against bed rails or gown
- Attempting to auscultate in a noisy room
- Interpreting chest hair sounds as adventitious lung sounds
- Auscultating only the "convenient" areas

Palpation of Chest Wall

ABN Findings & Interpretation

- Shift to "affected side": ↓ lung tissue (lobectomy, pneumonectomy)
- Shift to "unaffected side": ↑ pressure on lung (large pleural effusion)

Palpation for presence/absence of tracheal deviation.

ABN Findings & Interpretation *(Continued)*

■ Lack of symmetry between sides: area not moving equal to opposite side

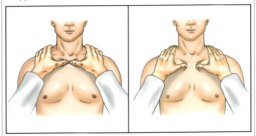

Palpation of upper lobe motion. (Redrawn from Cherniack RM, Cherniak L: Respiration in Health and Disease. 2nd ed. Philadelphia, WB Saunders, 1972. With permission from Elsevier.)

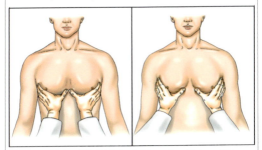

Palpation of right middle & left lingula lobe motion. (Redrawn from Cherniack RM, Cherniak L: Respiration in Health and Disease. 2nd ed. Philadelphia, WB Saunders, 1972. With permission from Elsevier.)

ABN Findings & Interpretation (Continued)

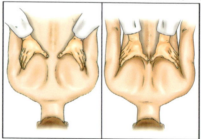

Palpation of lower lobe motion. (Redrawn from Cherniak RM, Cherniak L: Respiration in Health and Disease. 2nd ed. Philadelphia, WB Saunders, 1972. With permission from Elsevier.)

- ↓ ■ Muscle activity of scalenes: ↑ accessory muscle use; lack of diaphragmatic movement found in COPD, spinal cord injury, scarring, or improper breathing mechanics

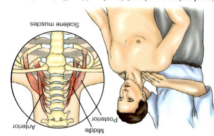

Palpation of scalene muscle activity w/breathing. (Redrawn from Cherniak RM, Cherniak L: Respiration in Health and Disease. 2nd ed. Philadelphia, WB Saunders, 1972. With permission from Elsevier.)

ABN Findings & Interpretation *(Continued)*

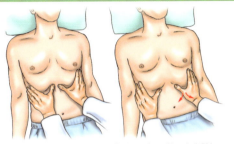

Palpation of diaphragmatic motion. (Redrawn from Cherniack RM, Cherniak L: Respiration in Health and Disease. 2nd ed. Philadelphia, WB Saunders, 1972. With permission from Elsevier.)

- Normally, palpation reveals uniform vibration throughout
- ↑ Vibration indicates secretions
- ↓ Fremitus indicates ↑ in air

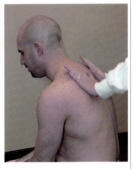

Palpation for fremitus (using heel of hand).

ABN Findings & Interpretation (Continued)

Rule out for angina pain:

■ ↓ Pain over bone indicates fracture; ↑ pain over muscle may be inflammation of muscles due to overuse or injury; ↑ discomfort w/deep inspiration or palpation is non-anginal

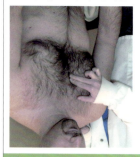

Palpation for chest wall pain or discomfort.

Assisted Breathing

Modes of O_2 Delivery

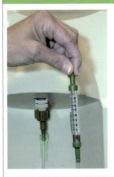

Modes: Flowmeter: w/bulk O_2 outlet
Indications: O_2 provided by institution from wall; use: acute care & high flow rates
Limitations/constraints: NOT portable; ↑ mobility w/tubing & nasal cannula or mask

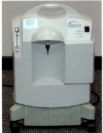

Modes: O_2 concentrator; H-cylinder
Indications: Contain 6900 L O_2; use: home or w/high flow rates
Limitations/constraints: Big: not portable

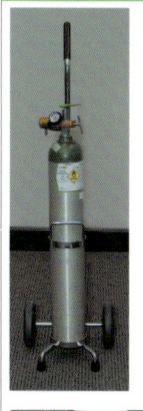

Modes: O$_2$ cylinders
Indications: Most widely used
Limitations/constraints: Heavy, wt:17 lb; hard to use & also has mobility problems; vol ↓ at high flow

Modes: Portable liquid O$_2$ unit
Indications: More lightweight for portable use
Limitations/constraints: Wt: 10 lb; empties fast w/high flow

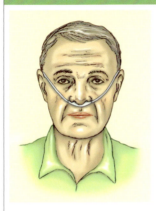

Modes: Nasal cannula
Indications: For use w/O₂ at flow rates of 1-6 L/min; provides FiO₂ of 24%-44%
Limitations/ constraints: No benefit if NOT breathing through nose

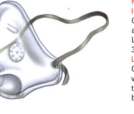

Modes: Simple mask
Indications: Delivery of O₂ over face w/humid air at ↑ flow rates (5-10 L/min); provides FiO₂ 35%-55%
Limitations/constraints: Claustrophobic w/mask, difficult to talk; best for mouth breather

Modes of O₂ Delivery (Continued)

Modes: Aerosol mask
Indications: For controlled %
of O₂ at flow rates > 10-12
L/min; FiO₂ 35%-100%
Limitations/constraints: Mask
not tolerated by pt for long
periods of time

Modes: Venturi mask
Indications: Provides greater flow of
gas w/use of room air through side
port (4-10 L/min); FiO₂ 24%-50%
Limitations/constraints: Mask not
tolerated by pt for long periods

Modes of O₂ Delivery *(Continued)*

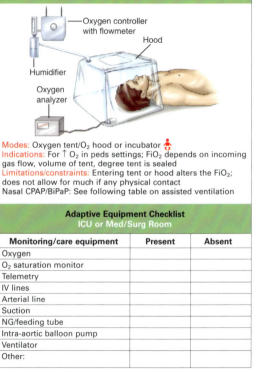

Oxygen controller with flowmeter

Hood

Humidifier

Oxygen analyzer

Modes: Oxygen tent/O₂ hood or incubator
Indications: For ↑ O₂ in peds settings; FiO₂ depends on incoming gas flow, volume of tent, degree tent is sealed
Limitations/constraints: Entering tent or hood alters the FiO₂; does not allow for much if any physical contact
Nasal CPAP/BiPaP: See following table on assisted ventilation

Adaptive Equipment Checklist
ICU or Med/Surg Room

Monitoring/care equipment	Present	Absent
Oxygen		
O₂ saturation monitor		
Telemetry		
IV lines		
Arterial line		
Suction		
NG/feeding tube		
Intra-aortic balloon pump		
Ventilator		
Other:		

Mechanical Ventilation/Assisted Ventilation	
Modes	**Indications**
Controlled vent: + pressure breaths at a set rate	To control rate, depth, & frequency of every breath
Assist or assist-control vent: + pressure breaths at set rate unless pt triggers machine w/neg inspir force < preset threshold force	Pt controls ventilations, but ↓ inspiration vol; used for postop care, weaning; to avoid ↑ peak airway pressure, & pt difficult to manage w/o sedation/paralyzing meds
IMV: preset rate, sponta-neous efforts +/− SIMV: mandatory breath initiated by spontaneous inspir effort	Pt can breathe spontaneously through ventilator circuit, but at preset intervals ventilator imposes mandatory breaths SIMV delivers a lower VT w/ higher airway pressure
PSV: patient's spontaneous vent efforts PLUS preset amt of pressure	Reduces work of breathing Used for postop care, weaning, to avoid high peak airway pres-sure, & pts difficult to manage w/o sedation/paralyzing drugs
Nasal CPAP	Treatment for obstructive sleep apnea
BiPap	Noninvasive vent: improves venti-lation & VS w/acute pulmonary edema; works more rapidly than CPAP
Vent: augmentation/ modifications 1. Inspiratory hold 2. PEEP 3. Expiratory retard 4. CPAP	1. Preset pressure or vol held for a set time before exhalation permitted. Used to ↓ atelectasis 2. Resistance after exhalation to keep alveoli open longer; recruits collapsed alveoli 3. Resistance applied to exhalation 4. Provides ↑ baseline pressure when pt breathing spontaneously

Cardiac Anatomy

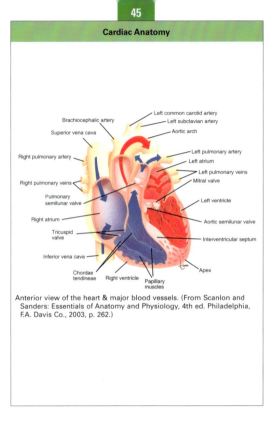

Anterior view of the heart & major blood vessels. (From Scanlon and Sanders: Essentials of Anatomy and Physiology, 4th ed. Philadelphia, F.A. Davis Co., 2003, p. 262.)

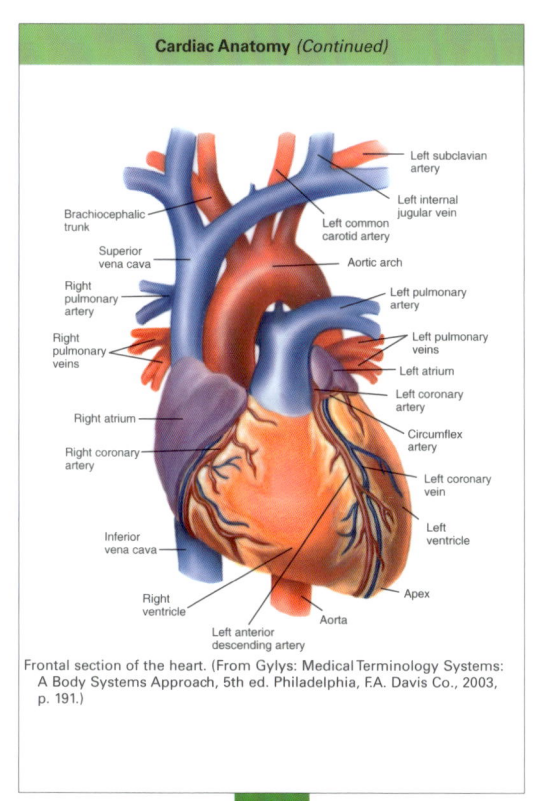

Frontal section of the heart. (From Gylys: Medical Terminology Systems: A Body Systems Approach, 5th ed. Philadelphia, F.A. Davis Co., 2003, p. 191.)

Ausculation of Heart Sounds

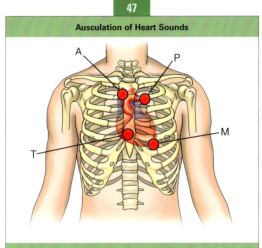

NL Heart Sounds

S_1 (lub of the lub-dub): associated w/closure of mitral & tricuspid valves; associated w/onset of systole
Loudest when auscultation at apex
S_2 (dub of the lub-dub): associated w/closure of pulmonic & aortic valves; associated w/onset of vent diastole
Loudest at aortic or pulmonic regions

ABN Heart Sounds

S$_3$ (an extra "dub" as in lub-dub-*dub*), heard after S$_2$: ausculta-tion w/bell of steth, best heard side-lying on left in mitral area. Sign of vent noncompliance or failure: vent gallop. In athlete: physiological NL sign

S$_4$ (extra sound before S$_1$: *la*-lub-dub)
Auscultation w/bell of steth: atrial gallop. Sign of ↑ resistance to vent filling. S$_4$ in: CAD, pulmonary disease, hypertensive heart disease, & post MI or CABG.

Murmurs
Grading: I-VI/VI:
- I/VI inaudible w/o steth
- IV-VI/VI very loud

Indicate backflow through valves
Between S$_1$ & S$_2$: systolic murmur. After S$_2$: diastolic

Pericardial Friction Rub
Squeaky/creaky leathery sound occurring w/each beat of heart. Indicates fluid in or inflammation of pericardial sac

Physiological Responses to Activity

	NL	ABN	Notes
HR	**Resting: 60-90 bpm**	**Resting:** <60 or >90 bpm	Athletes: RHR may be <60 Fever, anxiety, meds ↓ RHR Irregular at rest: check under-lying rhythm; see ECG section
	adult: ♀/♂ 50-100 bpm adolescent: 75-140 bpm child, 80-180 bpm infant	**Activity:** Rapid rate of ↑ or no ▲ w/ activity Irregular w/activity	
	Activity: Gradual rate of rise correlated w/intensity of activity ▲	**Steady state exercise:** Progressive ↑	
	Steady state exercise: No ▼		
	Rhythm should be regular		

Physiological Responses to Activity *(Continued)*

	NL	ABN	Notes
BP	**Resting**: Systolic <130 mm Hg; 🧍 70 mm Hg infant; 90 mm Hg child Diastolic <90 mm Hg; 55 mm Hg infant; 58 mm Hg child **Activity**: Systolic: progressive ↑ correlated w/ intensity of exercise Diastolic: +/− 10 mm Hg **Steady state exercise**: No ▲ in systolic or diastolic	**Resting**: Syst > 140 or Diast > 90 **Activity**: Rapid ↑ in systolic Blunted rate of rise w/↑ activity ↓ Systolic w/↑ activity Progressive ↑ in diastolic **Steady state exercise**: Progressive ↑	↓ in systolic w/▲ in position (sit to stand) is **orthostatic** ↓ w/activity: **exertional** hypotension Compare standing w/walking BP, NOT sitting to walking.
SpO₂	**Resting**: 98%-100% **Activity**: No ▲	**Resting**: <98% **Activity**: ↓ w/↑ activity	<90% is unstable Common to ↓ w/COPD
RR	**Adults Rest** 12-20 breaths/min 🧍**Peds Rest** 20-36 breaths/min **Activity**: ↑ related to amount of work	**Rest**:<12 or >20 for adults **Activity**: Anaerobic work: ↑ rapidly **Steady state exercise**: Breathing should adjust to exercise	Individuals ▲ breathing rate when being observed. Often counted while evaluating HR

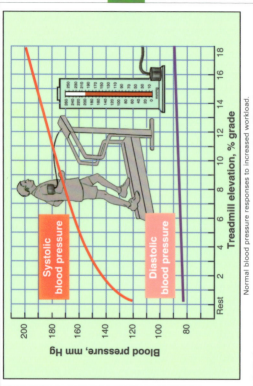

Normal blood pressure responses to increased workload.

Assess Responses to Activity

Activity	HR	BP	Symptoms	SpO$_2$	RPE
Supine					
Sit					
Stand					
Ambulation (include assistance needed, need for assistive device, feet walked)					
Performance of ADL					

RPE scale

6	
7	Very, very light
8	
9	Very light
10	
11	Fairly light
12	
13	Somewhat hard
14	
15	Hard
16	
17	Very hard
18	
19	Very, very hard

Borg scale. (Redrawn from Borg, GA: Psychological basis of physical exertion. Med Sci Sports Exerc 14:377, 1982.)

Assessment of Circulation

Arterial: Pulses

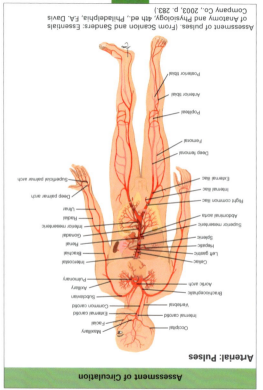

Occipital
Maxillary
Facial
External carotid
Internal carotid
Vertebral
Common carotid
Subclavian
Brachiocephalic
Axillary
Aortic arch
Pulmonary
Intercostal
Celiac
Left gastric
Hepatic
Splenic
Renal
Gonadal
Inferior mesenteric
Superior mesenteric
Abdominal aorta
Right common iliac
Internal iliac
External iliac
Brachial
Radial
Ulnar
Deep palmar arch
Superficial palmar arch
Deep femoral
Femoral
Popliteal
Anterior tibial
Posterior tibial

Assessment of pulses. (From Scanlon and Sanders: Essentials of Anatomy and Physiology, 4th ed., Philadelphia, FA. Davis Company Co., 2003, p. 283.)

Ankle Brachial Index:

Noninvasive test for evaluating peripheral arterial disease:

- Place pneumatic cuff around ankle above malleoli
- Place Doppler ultrasound probe over posterior tibial artery; measure pressure at this site
- Place Doppler probe over dorsalis pedis artery, measure pressure

NL pressures should differ no > 10 mm Hg

Pressure difference > 15 mm Hg suggests proximal occlusion or stenosis

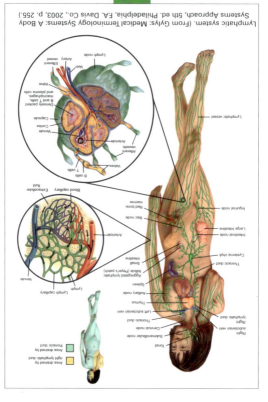

Lymphatic system. (From Gylys: Medical Terminology: A Body Systems Approach, 5th ed. Philadelphia, F.A. Davis Co., 2003, p. 255.)

Assessment of Edema

1+	Barely perceptible depression (pit)
2+	Easily identified depress (EID) rebounds w/in 15 sec
3+	EID rebounds to original w/in 15-30 sec
4+	EID rebounds >30 sec

Assessment of Angina & Dyspnea: Angina Scale

5-Grade Angina Scale	5-Grade Dyspnea Scale	10-Grade Angina/ Dyspnea Scale
0: No angina	0: No dyspnea	0: Nothing
1: Light, barely noticeable	1: Mild, noticeable	1: Very slight
	2: Mild, some difficulty	2: Slight
2: Moderate, bothersome	3: Moderate difficulty but can continue	3: Moderate
		4: Somewhat severe
3: Severe, very uncomfortable; pre-infarction pain	4: Severe difficulty, cannot continue	5: Severe
		6
		7: Very severe
		8
4: Most pain ever experienced; infarction pain		9
		10: Extremely severe: maximal

Cardiodiagnostics

Diagnostic Tests/Indications	Info Gathered from Tests	Precautions/Notes
CXR; eval of anatomic abnormalities & patho- logical process in lungs & chest wall	Lung size, heart size Integrity of ribs, sternum, clavicles, vascular markings Chronic vs. acute ▲ Lung fields: size, presence of fluid/ secretions, hyper/hypoinflation Presence of pleural fluid	AP films are often taken while pt is in bed; therefore pts often have hypoinflation due to a poor effort
ECG; eval of chest pain to determine if acute injury; eval of hypertrophy or old infarction (injury); eval of heart rhythm	Heart rhythm Old MI Vent/atrial hypertrophy Acute ischemia/injury/infarction conduction defects	Cannot *predict* ische- mia or infarction; stress test used to predict
Echocardiogram; eval of valve function &/or chamber sizes	Integrity, function of valves Chamber size, eval of pericardial sac	Noninvasive
Holter monitoring; eval of heart rhythm; eval of syncope	24-hour recording of rhythm of heart	Noninvasive
CT or MRI; ABN CXR showing nodule or mass	Enhanced pictures for interpretation of nodules or masses	

Cardiodiagnostics (Continued)

Diagnostic Tests/Indications	Info Gathered from Tests	Precautions/Notes
Stress testing Exercise stress Nuclear imaging w/exercise stress 2D/3D echo w/exercise stress Pharmacological stress (adenosine, dobut) Assess whether myocardial O_2 supply meets demand (assess for chest pain/coronary artery disease/ischemia) Determine aerobic capacity	Max VO_2, HR, BP response to activity, assessment of chest pain Assess ischemia Presence/absence of arrhythmias Limitation to exercise	Women have ↑ rates of false-positive & false-negative tests Need to have additional imaging w/stress testing (thallium, 2D/3D echo)
Coronary catheterization Chest pain, infarction	Blood flow through & integrity of coronary arteries Pressure changes across valves Estimated ejection fraction	Allergy to dye if pt has allergy to shellfish or iodine 24 hours of bedrest post cath through femoral artery

(Continued text on following page)

Cardiodiagnostics *(Continued)*

Diagnostic Tests/Indications	Info Gathered from Tests	Precautions/Notes
V/Q scans; rule out pulmonary emboli; especially in DVT	Gas distribution in lungs Regional ventilation matching of alveolar vent & pulm perfusion	
Bronchoscopy; obtain sputum sample for infection, malignancy; to clear viscous secretions not mobilized by pt	Direct visualization of inaccessible areas of bronchial tree	
PFT: classification of disease: obstructive vs restrictive; assess severity of disease or severity of acute illness	Integrity of airways Function of respiratory musculature Condition of lung tissues	

ECG/Arrhythmias

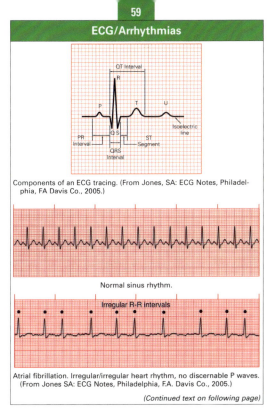

Components of an ECG tracing. (From Jones, SA: ECG Notes, Philadelphia, FA Davis Co., 2005.)

Normal sinus rhythm.

Atrial fibrillation. Irregular/irregular heart rhythm, no discernable P waves. (From Jones SA: ECG Notes, Philadelphia, F.A. Davis Co., 2005.)

(Continued text on following page)

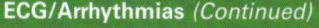

Premature ventricular contraction: uniform (same form) (wide, bizarre QRS, w/o P wave before).

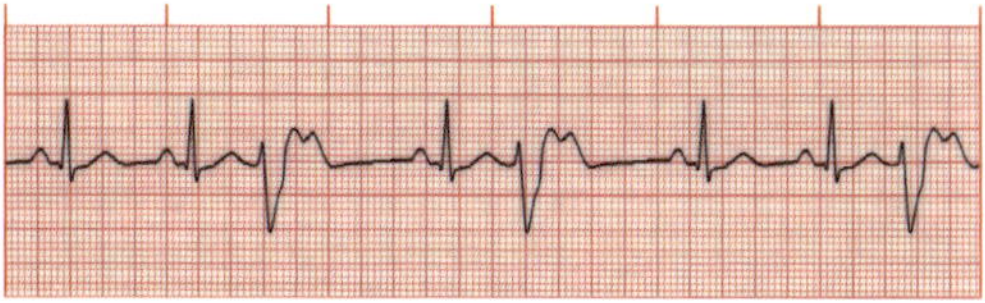

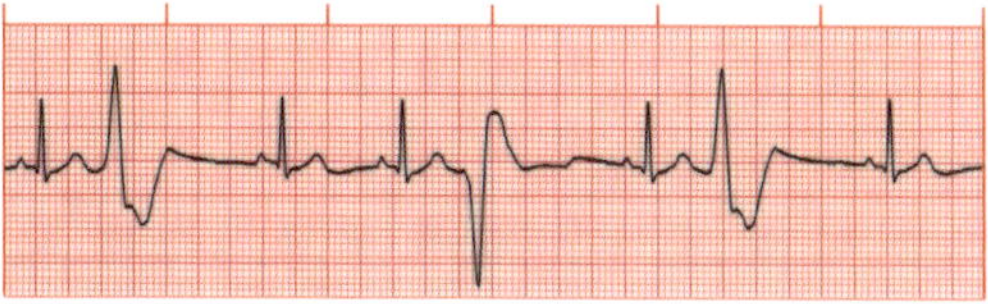

Premature ventricular contraction: multiform (different forms) (wide, bizarre QRS, w/o P wave before, & aberrant beats look different.) (From Jones SA: ECG Notes, Philadelphia, F.A. Davis Co., 2005.)

Atrial pacemaker spike   Ventricular pacemaker spike

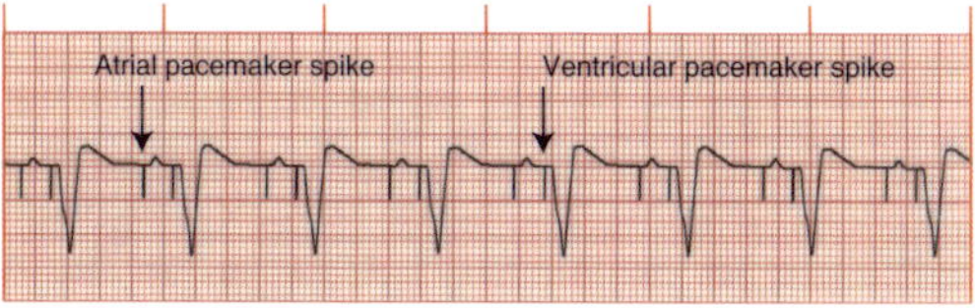

Dual-chamber pacemaker rhythm: atrial & ventricular vertical line before P wave, and/or QRS indicates pacemaker firing. (From Jones SA: ECG Notes, Philadelphia, F.A. Davis Co., 2005.)

Pulmonary Diagnostics

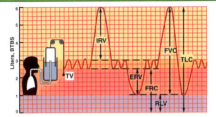

Lung Volume/Capacity	Definition	Average Values (ml) Men	Women
Tidal Volume (**TV**)	Volume inspired or expired per breath	600	500
Inspiratory Reserve Volume (**IRV**)	Maximum inspiration at end of tidal inspiration	3000	1900
Expiratory Reserve Volume (**ERV**)	Maximum expiration at end of tidal expiration	1200	800
Total Lung Capacity (**TLC**)	Volume in lungs after maximum inspiration	6000	4200
Residual Lung Volume (**RLV**)	Volume in lungs after maximum expiration	1200	1000
Forced Vital Capacity (**FVC**)	Maximum volume expired after maximum inspiration	4800	3200
Inspiratory Capacity (**IC**)	Maximum volume inspired following tidal expiration	3600	2400
Function Residual Capacity (**FRC**)	Volume in lungs after tidal expiration	2400	1800

Static measures of lung volumes. (Redrawn from McArdle WD, Katch FI, Katch VL: Exercise Physiology: Energy, Nutrition, and Human Performance, 4th ed. Williams & Wilkins, Baltimore, 1996.)

(Continued text on following page)

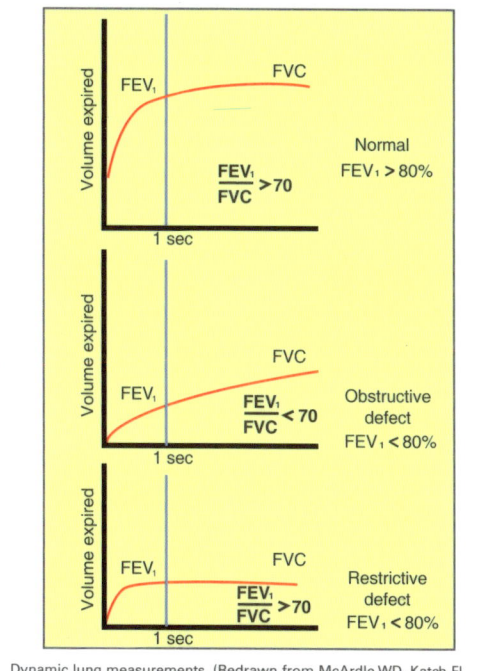

Dynamic lung measurements. (Redrawn from McArdle WD, Katch FI, Katch VL: Exercise Physiology: Energy, Nutrition, and Human Performance, 4th ed. Williams & Wilkins, Baltimore, 1996.)

Pulmonary Diagnostics *(Continued)*

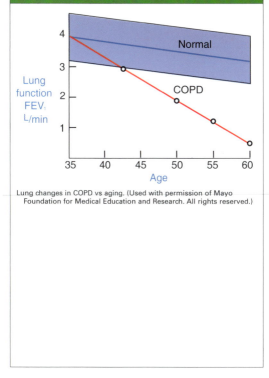

Lung changes in COPD vs aging. (Used with permission of Mayo Foundation for Medical Education and Research. All rights reserved.)

Exercise Assessments

6-Minute Walk Test

What it is:

Timed walk test to measure pt exercise endurance by observing distance covered in 6 min

How to do it:

Specific measured path (at least 100 ft in length); mark the walking surface at 10-ft intervals; chair avail every 50 ft

Pt walks at regular pace while therapist monitors SpO₂ & level of dyspnea for 6 min

Pt carries or wheels own O₂ & may rest when needs, but time continues to be counted during rests

Record distance, SpO₂, level of dyspnea, number of rests

Equipment needed:

Stopwatch

6-min walk documentation form

Steth & sphygmomanometer

Pulse oximetry

If needed, supplemental O₂ and/or telemetry

Treadmill Tests: Most Common Protocols

Bruce test: Used most often in hospitals for diagnostic purposes

Speed	Grade	Time
1.7 mph	10%	3 min
2.5 mph	12%	3 min
3.4 mph	14%	3 min
4.2 mph	16%	3 min
5.0 mph	18%	3 min

Balke test: Most often used for athletes

Start: 3.3 mph, 0%, grade ↑ 1% every min

Harbor/ramp test: Start walking at comfortable speed, ↑ grade each minute depending on fitness level

Talk Test

Talk test: Subjective measure of intensity of activity

Light: Individual can carry on full conversation while performing activity

Moderate: Minimal shortness of breath during conversation while performing activity

Vigorous: Individual w/ marked dyspnea; unable to converse while performing activity

Quick Screen

Evaluation/Screen	Results	NL/ABN
Heart sounds		
Lung sounds		
VS		
Symptoms		
Diagnostics: ECG		
Echo		
CXR		
PFT		
CXR		
Other		
Labs: Cholesterol/triglycerides		
CPK: MB, troponin, LDH-1		
Glucose, HbA1C		
BUN & creatinine		
Other ABN lab results?		
Meds: What are they & what are they used for?		

Exercise Assessment

Precautions w/Exercise

Abnormal Signs/Symptoms ▪ Abnormally high BP rise: systolic >240 mm Hg ▪ Diastolic >110 mm Hg ▪ Exercise hypotension (>10 mm Hg; systolic ↓ w/↑ activity)		
ABN HR response ▪ Rapid ↑ from rest in relation to activity ▪ Failure to ↑ w/↑ activity		
Symptoms of intolerance ▪ ↓ w/↑ activity (often indicates arrhythmia) ▪ Significant ↑ in angina ▪ Excessive dyspnea ▪ Excessive fatigue ▪ Mental confusion or dizziness ▪ Leg claudication		
Signs		
▪ Excessive fatigue		
▪ Mental confusion or dizziness		
▪ Leg claudication		
▪ Cold sweat		
▪ Ataxia		
▪ New heart murmur		
▪ Pallor		
▪ Auscultation of pulmonary rales		
▪ Onset of significant third heart sound (S₃)		
▪ Drop in SpO_2		
ECG		
▪ Serious arrhythmias (multifocal PVCs, couplets, triplets, etc.)		
▪ Second- or third-degree AV block		
▪ Acute ST changes		

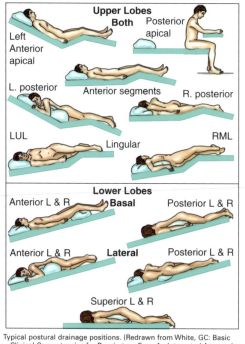

Upper Lobes
Both
Posterior apical

Left Anterior apical

L. posterior

Anterior segments

R. posterior

LUL

Lingular

RML

Lower Lobes
Basal

Anterior L & R

Posterior L & R

Anterior L & R

Lateral

Posterior L & R

Superior L & R

Typical postural drainage positions. (Redrawn from White, GC: Basic Clinical Competencies for Respiratory Care: An Integrated Approach. Albany, NY, Delmar Publishers, 1988.)

Exercise Prescription for Aerobic Exercise

Mode	Est ↓ VO₂ max w/exercise using large muscle groups over long time: walk, run, bike, etc
Intensity	Most commonly used: HR or RPE (see next table)
Frequency	Optimal is 3-5x per wk unless duration is <10-15 min; may work 7 x /wk if very poor exercise tolerance
Duration	Optimal: 20-30 min >30 min for wt loss programs <20 min for poor exercise tolerance: perform multiple short bouts

Heart Rate Methods for Determining Intensity

% HR max	Target HR (THR) should be 55%-75% of HR max
HR Reserve	THR = (HR max – HR rest) × (0.60-0.80) + HR rest
Deconditioned	Use lower % (40-60) or (0.40-0.60)

Caloric Cost of Exercise Estimation

(METs × 3.5 × body wt in kg)/200 = kcal/min

1 MET = 3.5 mL O₂/kg/min

Leisure Activities in METs

Activity	Mean	Range
Bowling	2.5	2–4
Conditioning exercise		3–8+
Dancing (aerobic)		6–9
Golf (cart use)		2–3
Running (12-min mile)	8.7	
Running (9-min mile)	11.2	
Skiing (downhill)		5–8
Soccer		5–12+
Tennis	6.5	4–9+

Indications for Referral

Indications for Referral	Suggested Referral Source
Elevated lipids (LDL, total chol, triglyc)	Dietitian, physician for lipid-lowering meds
Elevated blood glucose	Physician to evaluate for diabetes (possibly an endocrinologist), dietitian
↑ BMI	Dietitian, exercise program
Low albumin/prealbumin	Dietitian
ABN thyroid profile	Physician (possibly an endocrinologist)
Elevated BP	Physician for ↑ BP, meds, exercise program, dietitian
Continues to smoke	Smoking cessation program
Demonstrates anger/hostility easily	Psychologist/behavior specialist
Demonstrates s/s of depression	Psychologist/behavior specialist, physician for meds
Sedentary lifestyle	Exercise program
Elevated BMI or wt	Dietitian, exercise program

Special Considerations/Populations

Transplants (Heart & Lung)

Complications w/Heart & Lung Transplants

Immunosuppressive med side effects

- Renal dysfunction
- Hypertension
- Mood swings
- Skeletal muscle atrophy
- Osteoporosis
- ABN blood lipid profile

Acute rejection

Risk for opportunistic infections & malignancy

Accelerated graft coronary artery disease in heart transplant pts

Signs & Symptoms of Acute Rejection

Low-grade fever

↓ in resting blood pressure

Hypotension w/activities

Myalgias

Fatigue

↑ Exercise tolerance

Ventricular Arrhythmias

LVAD

Considerations for exercise testing & training in pts w/LVAD:

- Location of externalized drive line makes cycling & climbing stairs difficult
- HR response (palpated or from ECG) normal
- BP response variable due to fluid volume adjustment
- Consider skeletal muscle impairment if pt experienced long-standing CHF prior to LVAD

Responses to Activity in Cardiac Transplant Pts

Physiological Variables	Responses in Cardiac Transplant Pts
Rest HR	Elevated (>90 bpm)
Rest BP	Mildly elevated unless affected by meds
HR response to increasing activity	No △ first 5-10 min, followed by gradual rise w/activity
Peak HR	Slightly lower than normal (approx 150 bpm); often achieved during first few minutes of recovery
BP response to increasing activity	NL; peak BP lower than expected
Systemic vascular resistance	Generally elevated
Pulmonary vascular pressures	Generally elevated
Left vent systolic function (EF)	NL range at rest & w/exercise
Diastolic function (EDV)	Impaired: results in below normal ↑ in SV w/exercise
Skeletal muscle abnormalities	Greater reliance on anaerobic metabolic energy production
Ventilation	Efficiency is below normal ↑ VE/VCO$_2$: ↑ sense of SOB ↓ Rise in tidal volume w/exercise Diffusion impairment
Arterial-mixed venous O$_2$ content (a-vO$_2$ diff)	NL at rest, impaired w/exercise

Systems Affected by Diabetes

System	Impairments/Abnormalities	Implications for Rehab Professionals
Cardiovascular	↑ BP Impairment in circulation in extremities & small vessels Silent ischemia/silent MI	Monitor BP at rest & w/activity Evaluate any wounds Monitor symptoms w/activity; look for SOB: NOT angina
Endocrine	↑ Cholesterol ↑ Triglycerides	Evaluate lab results; referral to control lipids
Integumentary	Impaired healing due to impaired circulation	Evaluate skin; assess post-surgical scars/incisions
Nervous	■ Peripheral neuropathies ■ → Sensation in hands & feet ■ → Sensation of chest pain ■ Autonomic neuropathies ■ Orthostatic hypotension ■ ABN VS responses	■ Instruct in skin checks, foot care & good footwear ■ SOB = angina in diabetics/may not perceive typical angina ■ Monitor VS w/all activities
Ophthalmic	■ Retinopathies: poor vision	■ Assess visual
Renal	■ Renal artery disease: impaired function of glomerulus, impaired filtering	■ Rule out kidney problems by evaluating labs (creat & BUN)

Signs/Symptoms of Hypoglycemia

Adrenergic Signs/Symptoms: Weakness, sweating, tachycardia, palpitations, tremor, nervousness, irritability, tingling mouth & fingers, hunger, nausea, vomiting

Neuroglucopenic Signs/Symptoms: Headache, hypothermia, visual disturbances, mental dullness, confusion, amnesia, seizures, coma

Exercise Considerations for Diabetics

- Type of insulin used
- Onset of effect of insulin
- Peak effect of insulin
- Length of insulin effect

Injection site
Time between insulin taken & onset of exercise
Time between exercise & last meal
See Tab 7 for Insulins Weight Management

Equations for Prediction of Basal Metabolic Rate Based on Wt

Males		Females	
Age (yr)	kcal/day	Age (yr)	kcal/day
18-30	15.3 × wt in kg + 679	18-31	14.7 × wt in kg + 496
30-60	11.6 × wt in kg + 879	30-61	8.7 × wt in kg + 829
>60	13.5 × wt in kg + 487	>61	10.5 × wt in kg + 596

Primary Components of Healthy Wt Loss Program

Total Calories	**Women: no fewer than 1200 cal/day** **Men: no fewer than 1500 cal/day**
Fat	<30% cal, ↓ sat fat & trans fatty acids
Protein	20%-25% cal, no fewer than 75 g/day
Carbo	50% of cal, not <5 servings of fruits & vegetables ↑ Simple sugars, ↓ complex sugars (starches)
Dietary Fiber	20-30 g/day from food sources
Water	Not less than 1 L/day
Alcohol	Limit intake

Pts w/Pacemakers, ICDs, & IABP

Invasive Monitoring or Device	Implications for Rehab Professionals
Pacemakers ■ Fixed rate (FR) ■ Demand (D) ■ A-V sequential	Identify type of pacemaker FR: HR will not ↑ w/activity; will make heart contract at SET HR D: HR will ↑ w/activity Pacemaker initiates vent contraction when HR drops below a set rate A-V: Most common pacemaker; atria stimulated to depolarize, then ventricles Left UE ROM above shoulder restricted for 24-72 hr after implant
■ **ICD**	Corrects life-threatening arrythmias. Used in high risk for sudden death pop. Left UE ROM above shoulder restricted for 24-72 hr after implant.

Pts w/Pacemakers, ICDs, & IABP *(Continued)*	
Invasive Monitoring or Device	**Implications for Rehab Professionals**
■ IABP	Used to ↑ diastolic BP & ↑ coronary blood flow. Use: hemodynamically unstable pt. Hip flexion kept <70°. OOB contraind. Only ROM & bed mobility

Disease Management Outcomes

Cardiac Rehabilitation Outcomes

Behavioral Outcomes: Diet: compliance w/diet, wt management, exercise: compliance w/exercise program, smoking cessation, stress reduction, recognize signs/symptoms, medical management

Clinical Outcomes: Wt/BMI, BP, lipids, functional capacity, blood nicotine levels, O_2 saturation, symptom mgmnt, psychosocial: return to vocation/leisure, psychological status, medical utilization, hospitalizations, meds, physician/ER visits

Health Outcomes: Morbidity, future events: MI, CABG, angioplasty, new angina, serious arrhythmias, mortality, QOL, tools: generic or disease-specific

Pulmonary Rehabilitation Outcomes

Behavior Domain: Smoking cessation, breathing retraining, coping strategies, bronchial hygiene, med adherence, supplemental O_2 use, pacing techniques, energy conservation, sexual function, adherence to diet

Clinical Domain: Fatigue, depression/anxiety, physical performance measures, exercise duration, exercise performance on a walk test, exertional dyspnea, dyspnea w/daily activities

Health Domain: Mortality, health-related QOL, morbidity, no. rehospitalizations, time between physician visits for illness, health care utilization, no. ER visits

Service Domain: Pt satisfaction

Evaluation Notes for Practice Pattern

Patterns	Included Diagnoses	Prognosis
6A: Primary prevention & risk reduction for CV/pulmonary disorders	Diabetes, obesity, hypertension, sedentary lifestyle, smoking, hypercholesterolemia, hyperlipidemia	Pt will ↓ risk for CV/pulmonary disorders w/therapeutic exercise, aerobic conditioning, functional training, & lifestyle modification
6B: Impaired aerobic cap/endur associated w/ deconditioning	AIDS, cancer, CV disorders, chronic systems failure, inactivity, multisystem impairments, musculoskeletal disorders, neuromuscular disorders, pulmonary disorders	In 6-12 wk, pt will demonstrate optimal aerobic cap/endur & >established level of function in home, work, community, & leisure environs
6C: Impaired ventilation, resp/gas exchange, & aerobic cap/endur associated w/airway clearance dysfunction	Acute lung disorders, Acute/chronic O₂ dependency, bone marrow/stem cell transplants, cardiothoracic surgery, △ in baseline breath sounds, △ in baseline CXR, COPD, frequent/recurring pulmonary infection, solid-organ transplants, tracheostomy or microtracheostomy	In 12-16 wk, pt will demonstrate optimal vent, resp. and/or gas exchange, & aerobic cap/endur & >est level of function in home, work, community, & leisure environs within the context of the impairment

Evaluation Notes for Practice Pattern (Continued)

Patterns	Included Diagnoses	Prognosis
6D: Impaired aerobic cap/ aerobic cap/aerobic cap/endur associated w/CV pump dys-function or failure	Angioplasty/atherectomy, AV block, cardiogenic shock, cardiomyopathy, cardiothoracic surgery, complex vent >est level of function in home, work, community, & leisure environs within context of impairment, functional limits, & disabilities arrhythmia, complicated myocardial infarction (failure), uncomplicated myocardial infarction (dysfunction), congenital cardiac abnormalities, coronary artery disease, ↓ ejection fraction (<50%), diabetes, exercise-induced myocardial ischemia, hyper-tensive heart disease, nonmalignant arrhythmias, valvular heart disease	In 6-12 wk, pt w/CV pump dysfunction will show opt aerobic cap/endur & >est level of function in home, work, community, & leisure environs within context of impairment, functional limits, & disabilities In 8-16 wk, pt w/CV pump failure will show optimal aerobic cap/endur (etc.)
6E: Impaired ventilation & resp/gas exchange associated w/ventilatory pump dys-function or failure	Elevated diaphragm + volume loss on CXR, neuromuscular disorders, partial/complete diaphragmatic paralysis, poliomyelitis, pulmonary fibrosis, restrictive lung disease, severe kyphoscoliosis, spinal/cere-bral neoplasm, spinalcord injury	In 3-6 wk, pt w/vent pump dysfunction or reversible vent pump failure will show opt independence w/vent & resp/gas exchange & > level of function in home, work, community, & leisure environs, within context of impair-ment, functional limits, & disabilities In 9-10 wk, pt w/prolonged, severe, or chronic vent pump failure will demonstrate optimal independence w/vent & resp/gas exchange & (etc.) (Continued text on following page)

Evaluation Notes for Practice Pattern (Continued)

Patterns	Included Diagnoses	Prognosis
6F: Impaired vent & resp/gas exchange associated w/respiratory failure	ABN CXR, acute neuromuscular dysfunction, ARDS, ABN alveolar to arterial oxygen tension differences, asthma, cardiothoracic surgery, COPD, inability to maintain O_2 tension w/supplemental O_2, multisystem failure, pneumonia, pre/post lung transplant or rejection, rapid rise in arterial CO_2 at rest or w/ activity, sepsis, thoracic or multisystem trauma	Within 72 hr, pt w/*acute reversible resp failure* will demonstrate optimal independence w/vent & resp/gas exchange & > established level of function in home, work, community, & leisure environs Within 3 wks, pt w/*prolonged resp failure* will demonstrate optimal indep w/vent, (etc.) In 4–6 wk, pt w/*severe or chronic resp failure* will demonstrate optimal indep w/vent, (etc.)
6G: Impaired vent, resp/gas exchange, & aerobic cap/endur associated w/respiratory failure in the neonate	ABN thoracic surgeries, apnea & bradycardia, bronchopulmonary dysphasia, congenital anomalies, hyaline membrane disease, meconium aspiration syndrome, neurovascular disorders, pneumonia, rapid desaturation w/movement or crying	In 6–12 mo, pt will demonstrate optimal vent, resp/gas exchange, & aerobic cap/endur & the >est level of age-appropriate function

Evaluation Notes for Practice Pattern (Continued)

Patterns	Included Diagnoses	Prognosis
6H: Impaired circulation & anthropometric dimensions associated w/ lymphatic system disorders	AIDS, cellulitis, filariasis, infection/sepsis, lymphedema, postradiation, reconstructive surgery, reflex sympathetic dystrophy, status post lymph node dissection, trauma	Within 1-8 wk, pt w/ *mild lymphedema (<3 cm differential between affected limb & unaffected limb)* will demonstrate optimal circ. & anthrop. dimensions & >established level of function in home, work, community, & leisure environs within context of the impairment, functional limits, & disabilities Within 1-8 wk, pt w/ *moderate lymphedema (3-5 cm differential)* will demonstrate optimal circ., etc. Within 8 wk, pt w/ *severe lymphedema (5 plus cm differential)* will demonstrate optimal circ, etc.

Musculoskeletal Assessment

Quick Screen

Upper Quarter Screening Exam

1. Posture assessment
2. Active ROM cervical spine
3. Passive overpressures if symptom-free
4. Passive muscle tests cervical spine (rotation C-1)
5. Resisted shoulder elevation (C2, 3, 4)
6. Resisted shoulder abduction (C5)
7. Active shoulder flexion & rotations
8. Resisted elbow flexion (C-6)
9. Resisted elbow extension (C-7)
10. Active ROM elbow
11. Resisted wrist flexion (C-7)
12. Resisted wrist extension (C-6)
13. Resisted thumb extension (C-8)
14. Resisted finger abduction (T-1)
15. Babinski's reflex test for UMN

Lower Quarter Screening Exam*

1. Postural assessment
2. Active forward, backward, & lateral bending of lumbar spine
3. Toe raises (S-1)
4. Heel walking (L-4, 5)
5. Active rotation of lumbar spine
6. Overpressure if symptom-free
7. Straight leg raise (L-4, 5, S-1)
8. Sacroiliac spring test
9. Resisted hip flexion (L-1, 2)
10. Passive ROM to hip
11. Resisted knee extension (L-3, 4)
12. Knee flexion, extension, medial, & lateral tilt
13. Femoral nerve stretch
14. Babinski's reflex test for UMN

*Adapted from Cyriax & Cyriax: Illustrated Manual of Orthop Med, ed 2. Butterworth, 1993.

Pain Assessment
Ransford Pain Assessment

/ / / Stabbing	x x x Burning
000 Pins/needles	=== Numbness

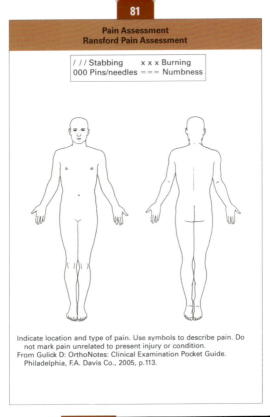

Indicate location and type of pain. Use symbols to describe pain. Do not mark pain unrelated to present injury or condition.

From Gulick D: OrthoNotes: Clinical Examination Pocket Guide. Philadelphia, F.A. Davis Co., 2005, p.113.

Ransford Scoring System

The following are scored 2 points each for pain in:

	Points
■ Total leg	
■ Front of leg	
■ Anterior tibial	
■ Back of leg & knee	
■ Circumferential thigh	
■ Lateral whole leg	
■ Bilateral foot	
■ Circumferential foot	
■ Anterior knee & ankle	
■ Throughout whole leg	
■ Entire abdomen	

Additional Points

■ Drawings w/expansion or magnification of pain (1-2 points)	
■ Back pain radiating into iliac crest, groin, & anterior perineum	
■ Pain drawn outside of diagram	
■ Additional explanations, circles, lines, arrows (1 point each)	
■ Painful areas drawn in (1 point for small area, 2 points for large)	

Total Score

Interpretation

A score of 3 or more points is thought to represent pain perception that may be influenced by psychological factors.

Pain Questions

1. Where is your pain? _____
2. What brings pain on? _____
3. What takes pain away? _____
4. Does pain travel to different areas? _____
5. Does pain always feel the same? _____
6. When is pain worst? _____
7. When is pain least? _____
8. Do you have joint swelling? _____
9. Do you have pain w/muscle spasms? _____
10. Do you have any numbness, tingling, burning pain? _____
11. Do you have hot or cold sensations with your pain? _____

Medical Screening for Possible Systemic Involvement: Associated Symptoms w/Pain

If "yes" to any of the following, check for presence of these symptoms bilaterally (indicates referral to physician)

_____ Blumberg's sign: rebound tenderness/pain on palpation
_____ Burning
_____ Difficulty breathing
_____ Difficulty swallowing
_____ Dizziness
_____ Heart palpitations
_____ Headache or visual changes
_____ Hoarseness
_____ Insidious onset w/no known mechanism of injury
_____ Nausea
_____ Numbness and/or tingling
_____ No change in symptoms despite positioning or rest
_____ Night sweats
_____ Pigmentation or changes, edema, rash, weakness, numbness, tingling, burning
_____ Psoas test for pelvic pathology; SLR to 30° in supine & hip flex resisted
  ■ + test for pelvic inflammation or infection/abdominal pain
  ■ − test indicates hip/back pain

Medical Screening *(Continued)*

____ Symptoms persist beyond expected healing time
____ Symptoms out of proportion to injury
____ Throbbing
____ Unexplained wt loss, pallor, bowel/bladder changes
____ Violent left shoulder pain (may be referred from spleen)
____ Vomiting
____ Weakness

Range of Motion for Adults (AAOS)*

Joint/Motion	Range (in degrees)
Cervical spine – flexion	0– 45
– extension	0– 45
– lateral flexion	0– 45
– rotation	0– 60
Shoulder – flexion	0–180
– extension	0– 60
– abduction	0–180
– internal rotation	0– 70
– external rotation	0– 90
– horizontal adduction	0–135
Elbow – flexion	0–150
Radioulnar – pronation	0– 80
– supination	0– 80
Wrist – flexion	0– 80
– extension	0– 70
– radial deviation	0– 20
– ulnar deviation	0– 30

Range of Motion for Adults (AAOS)* *(Continued)*

Joint/Motion	Range (in degrees)
Thoracolumbar/lumbosacral – flexion	0–80 (or 4 inches)
– extension	0–(20–30)
– lateral flex	0–35
– rotation	0–45
Hip – flexion	0–120
– extension	0–30
– abduction	0–45
– adduction	0–30
– internal rotation	0–45
– external rotation	0–45
Knee – flexion	0–135
Ankle – plantarflexion	0–50
– dorsiflexion	0–20
Subtalar – inversion	0–35
– eversion	0–15

*AAOS = American Academy of Orthopedic Surgeons

Common End Feels w/Passive ROM

Capsular	Slow w/a building up of resistance (like stretching a belt; e.g., knee ext)
Ligamentous	Like capsular, but a little harder: solid stop w/o pain
Soft tissue approximation	Feels like a painful squeeze: movement stopped by contact w/adjacent soft tissue
Bone on bone	Hard, sudden stop
Muscle tightening/elastic	Feel muscle reaction similar to other soft tissue, but hold-relax alters it: muscle tightness limits motion

(Continued text on following page)

Common End Feels w/Passive ROM *(Continued)*	
Springlike	Muscle reaction is equal & opposite to pressure given, e.g., spring
Empty	Pt will not allow end feel due to pain

Strength Assessment (Muscle Performance) Grading System*

Grade	Definition
5 (NL)	Completes full ROM against gravity; maintains end-range against maximal resistance
4 (good)	Completes full ROM against gravity; maintains end-range against strong resistance
3+ (fair+)	Completes full ROM against gravity; maintains end-range against mild resistance
3 (fair)	Completes full ROM against gravity; unable to maintain end-range against any resistance
2 (poor)	Completes full ROM in a gravity-eliminated position
1 (trace)	Observable or palpated contractile activity in muscle w/o movement
0 (none)	No activity detected in muscle

*Hislop and Montgomery grading

Segmental motor innervation: Upper extremity

	C4	C5	C6	C7	C8	T1
Shoulder	--- Supraspinatus ---					
	---Teres minor---					
		----Deltoid----				
		----Infraspinatus----				
		---- Subscapularis ----				
		---- Teres major----				
Arm		---- Biceps----				
		----Brachialis----				
		------Coracobrachialis---				
			--------Triceps brachialis ---		
			----- Anconeus ---		
Forearm		--Supinator longus-				
		---- Supinator brevis ----				
			--Extensor carpi radialis ---		
			--Pronator teres---		
			-Flexor carpi radialis		
				-- Flexor pollicis longus ---	
				·Extensor pollicis brevis	
				Extensor pollicis longus	
				--- Extensor digitorum longus	
				--- Extensor indicis proprius	
				----·Extensor carpi ulnaris	
				----·Extensor digiti quinti	
				--- Flexor digitorum sublimis ---	
				--Flexor digitorum profundus-	
				---- Pronator quadratus ---	
				--- Flexor carpi ulnaris ------	
				--·Palmaris longus ----	
				Abductor pollicis brevis---	
Hand				--·Flexor pollicis brevis--	
				Opponens pollicis·-	
				--·Flexor digiti quinti-	
				-Opponens digiti quinti-	
				Adductor pollicis --	
				·Palmaris brevi ----	
				Abductor digiti quinti	
				---·Lumbricales----	
				---·Interossei------	

Segmental motor innervation: Lower extremity

	L1	L2	L3	L4	L5	S1	S2

Hip

- Iliopsoas
- Tensor fasciae latae
- Gluteus medius
- Gluteus minimus
- Gracilis
- Quadratus femoris
- Gemellus inferior
- Gemellus superior
- Gluteus maximus
- Obturator internus
- Piriformis

Thigh

- Sartorius
- Pectineus
- Adductor longus
- Quadratus femoris
- Gracilis
- Adductor brevis
- Obturator externus
- Adductor magnus
- Adductor minimus
- Semimembranosus
- Semitendinosus
- Biceps femoris

Leg

- Tibialis anticus
- External hallucis longus
- Popliteus
- Plantaris
- External digitorum longus
- Soleus
- Gastrocnemius
- Peroneus longus
- Peroneus brevis
- Tibialis posterior
- Flexor digitorum longus
- Flexor hallucis longus

Feet

- Extensor digitorum brevis
- Extensor hallucis brevis
- Flexor digitorum brevis
- Abductor hallucis
- Flexor hallucis brevis
- Lumbricales
- Adductor hallucis
- Abductor digiti quinti
- Flexor digiti quinti
- Opponens digiti quinti
- Quadratus plantaris
- Interossei

	Joint Integrity Testing	
Joint	**Ligament/ Joint Test**	**Description**
Shoulder	Apprehension	Abduct shoulder to 90° & ER to tolerance
	AC shear	AP compression of AC joint
	CC test	Side-lying, UE behind back, abducted inferior angle of scapula (conoid) or abducted vertebral border of scapula (trapezoid)
Elbow	Medial & lateral collateral	Varus force = LCL/RCL Valgus force = MCL/UCL
Wrist & Hand	Collaterals of wrist & digits	Varus force =LCL/RCL Valgus force = MCL/UCL
Hip: Peds	1. Ortolani's test 2. Barlow's test	1. Supine; one hip abducted & thigh raised w/fingers to reduce hip; other hand stabilizes pelvis 2. Supine; thumb on inner thigh & hip adducted w/ longitudinal pressure on thigh
Adult	1. Trendelenburg's test 2. Scour	1. Standing: on leg w/opposite limb raised: test is for weak gluteus medius if pelvis falls 2. IR/ER hip w/abduction/ adduction while applying compress force femur down to test for labral tear

(Continued text on following page)

Joint Integrity Testing (Continued)

Joint	Ligament/ Joint Test	Description
Knee	Collaterals	Varus stress for LCL Valgus stress for MCL
	Lachman's test	Supine, knee flexed 30°, proximal tibia moved forward to test ACL
	Posterior drawer	Supine, hip flexed 45°, knee flexed 90°, grasp back of proximal tibia, tibia drawn back on femur to test PCL
Ankle	Anterior drawer	Grasp postcalcaneus & move anterior on tibia/ fibula to assess for ATF laxity
	Talar tilt	Apply varus stress on talus using calcaneus & plantarflexion to test ATF, in neutral (CF), & dorsiflexion (PTF)
	Squeeze	Supine two-knee extension; compress tibia/fibula together from proximal (at knee) distally to assess for syndesmotic sprain

Most Common Knee Joint Stability Tests

Vertebral Motion Related to Facet Function

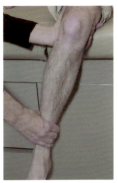

Valgus stress test.

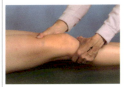

Lachman's test.

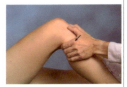

Posterior drawer.

Spinal Mobility

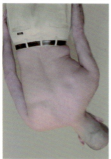

(A) Forward bending motion. Facets open.

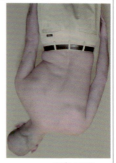

(B) Backward bending motion. Facets closed.

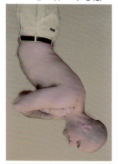

(C) Side bending right motion. Right facet closes, left facet opens.

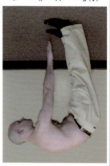

(D) Side bending left motion. Right facet opens, left facet closes.

Task	Level of Impairment			
	Intact	Min	Mod	Max
Perception				
Attention				
Cognition				
Arousal				
Sensation				
Tone				
Mov't patterns				
Sitting balance				
Standing balance				

Motor Control

Courtesy of Dawn Gulick.

Posture Assessment

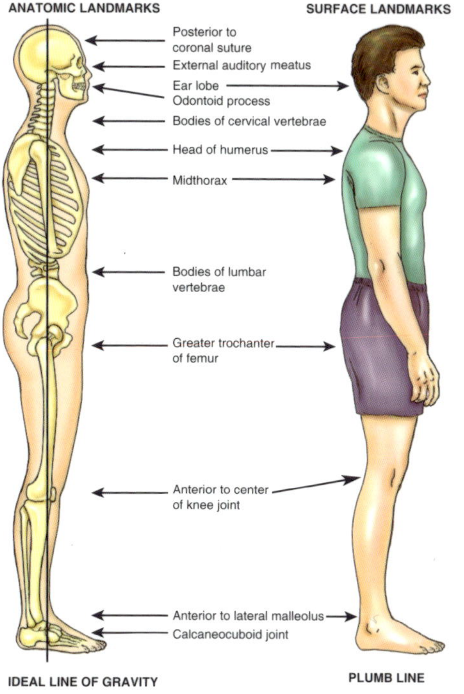

ANATOMIC LANDMARKS

SURFACE LANDMARKS

Posterior to
coronal suture

External auditory meatus

Ear lobe
Odontoid process

Bodies of cervical vertebrae

Head of humerus

Midthorax

Bodies of lumbar
vertebrae

Greater trochanter
of femur

Anterior to center
of knee joint

Anterior to lateral malleolus

Calcaneocuboid joint

IDEAL LINE OF GRAVITY

PLUMB LINE

Lateral view.

ANATOMIC LANDMARKS

SURFACE LANDMARKS

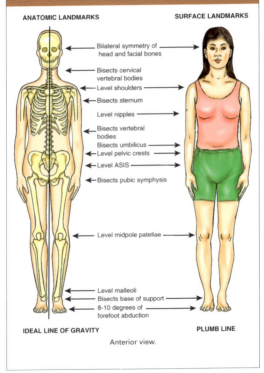

Bilateral symmetry of head and facial bones

Bisects cervical vertebral bodies

Level shoulders

Bisects sternum

Level nipples

Bisects vertebral bodies

Bisects umbilicus

Level pelvic crests

Level ASIS

Bisects pubic symphysis

Level midpole patellae

Level malleoli

Bisects base of support

8-10 degrees of forefoot abduction

IDEAL LINE OF GRAVITY

PLUMB LINE

Anterior view.

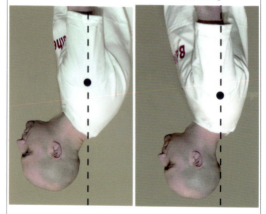

Kyphosis.

Forward head.

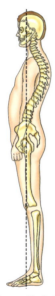

Increased lordosis.

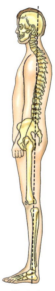

Flat back.

Postural Variations (Continued)

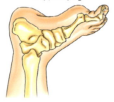

Supinated foot.

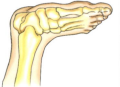

Pronated foot.

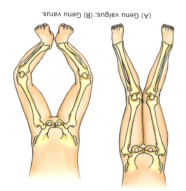

(A) Genu valgus; (B) Genu varus.

Postural Deformity Term	Common Problems Associated w/Deformity
Forward head position	Upper cervical pain, headache; progresses to spinal deformities: e.g., thoracic kyphosis, & ↓ lumbar lordosis
Cervical/thoracic kyphosis	Upper cervical pain, headache, abducted scapulae, stretched & weak posterior trunk muscles, shortened anterior musculature
Scapular winging Scapular elevation/ depression Scapular retraction	Weak UEs, weak scapular stabilizers (serratus, mid & lower trapezius) Muscle spasms in upper thoracic area
Increased lumbar lordosis	Hypermobile in extension, hypomobile in flexion, sheer stresses to L4, L5 & L5, S1; ↓ strength of abdominal muscles, shortened hip flexors: ↑ risk of disk disease
Decreased lumbar lordosis	May lead to disk disease
Genu valgus (a) Genu varus (b)	(a) Leads to medial knee & ankle pain & lateral hip pain (b) Lateral knee & ankle pain
Pes planus (flat foot)	↑ Valgus stress on knees; ABN stress on joints of foot
Pes cavus (high arch)	↑ Stress on all LE structures & spine

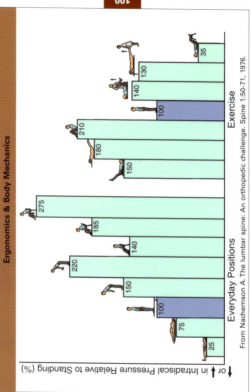

Ergonomics & Body Mechanics

% in Intradiscal Pressure Relative to Standing (%)

Everyday Positions

Exercise

From Nachemson A. The lumbar spine: An orthopedic challenge. Spine 1:50-71, 1976.

Prevention of Neck & Back Injuries

Activities: Sleeping
Correct Positions: Pillow should keep spine straight & neck & lumbar back in neutral

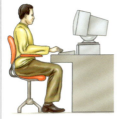

Activities: Sitting at work
Correct Positions: Desk, chair, & monitor adjusted so monitor is eye level
Use armrest
Sit w/spine against back of chair
Knees slightly lower than hips
Use footstool
Correct Positions: Move fingers only
Maintain a straight-wrist position
Consider wrist splints to decrease work on wrists

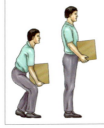

Activities: Lifting heavy objects
Correct Positions: Keep object close to your center of gravity
Contract abdominals
Use legs & hips to lift; not neck & back

Gait, Locomotion, & Balance		
Observational Gait Analysis:	**NL**	**ABN**
Reciprocal arm swing		
Rotation of shoulders & thorax		
Pelvic rotation		
Hip flexion & extension (min flexion: 30°)		
Knee flexion & extension (min flexion: 40°; 70° for stairs)		
Ankle dorsiflexion & plantar flexion (min 15° dorsiflexion, 15° plantarflexion)		
Step length (right = left)		
Stride length (NL = 70-82 cm or 27-32 in)		
Heel rise		
Pre-swing		
Cadence (NL = 90-120 steps/min)		
Pelvic rotation		
Pelvic list		
Hip rotation & abduction-adduction		
Knee rotation & abduction/adduction		
Degree of toeing-out		
Base of support measurement		
Subtalar movement		

Abnormalities of Gait

Phase	Deviations	Causes/Problems
Both	Antalgic gait: ■ Decrease in duration of stance of affected limb ■ Lack of wt shift over stance limb ■ Decrease in swing phase of uninvolved side	Pain in lower limb or pelvic region Limited ROM or strength in one extremity
Both	Trendelenburg's gait: Pelvis drops on unaffected side during single-limb support of side of weakness, or lurching gait w/laterally flexing of trunk over affected limb	Gluteus medius weakness
Stance: heel strike	Quick moving of trunk posteriorly at initial contact w/ground, allowing for upright posture to be maintained	Paralysis or weakness of gluteus maximus
Stance	When shorter limb makes contact w/ground: pelvis drops laterally, longer limb joints show exaggerated flexion or circumduction	Leg length discrepancy
Stance	Lengthening of uninvolved limb (hip hiking) to achieve swing-through of affected limb	Joint hypomobility of hip or knee flexion
Stance	Forward bending of trunk w/rapid plantar flexion to create extension	Inability of quadriceps to contract

(Continued text on following page)

Abnormalities of Gait (Continued)

Phase	Deviations	Causes/Problems
Stance	Diminished stance phase of affected side & smaller step length on unaffected side; no true propulsion because of weakness	Weakness or paralysis of ankle plantar flexors
	Increased lumbar lordosis & backward bending of trunk	Hip flexion contracture
	Early heel rise during terminal stance; knee hyperextension at midstance & forward bending of trunk w/hip flexion	Plantar flexion contracture
Swing	Difficulty in initiating swing-through; rotates limb externally at hip, using adductors to achieve swing-through.	Weakness of psoas muscle
	Steppage gait; increased hip & knee flexion to compensate for dropfoot	Lack of ankle dorsiflexion
	Foot slap during ground contact	Weak anterior tibialis
	Excessive dorsiflexion of ankle during late swing phase to early stance of uninvolved limb; involved limb: early heel rise in terminal stance	Knee flexion contracture

Gait Training w/ Assistive Devices

Gait Pattern: Four-point pattern for bilateral assistive device
Description: One crutch, contralateral lower limb, other crutch, then other lower limb

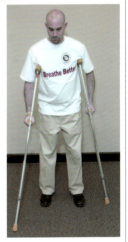

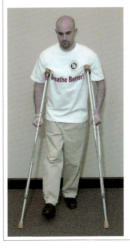

Gait Pattern: Three-point pattern using unilateral assistive device
Description: Assistive device on opposite side of involved lower limb. Start: assistive device advanced, involved lower limb, then uninvolved lower limb
Walker forward first, then involved limb, then uninvolved limb

Gait Pattern: Two-point pattern: assistive device & involved lower limb move together

Description: Assistive device & involved lower limb move forward, then uninvolved lower limb forward

Walker forward first, non-weightbearing involved limb forward, then uninvolved limb

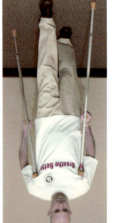

Gait Pattern: Stair climbing

Description: Ascend stairs w/uninvolved leg first, followed by involved leg & assistive device

Descend stairs w/assistive device & involved leg first, then uninvolved leg

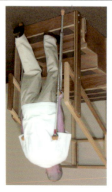

Self Care & Home Management Assessment

Task	Level of Assistance Requires				
	Independent	Supervised	Minimal	Moderate	Maximal
Bed Mobility - Roll side to side	I	S	Min	Mod	Max
Move up & down in bed	I	S	Min	Mod	Max
Supine to sit/sit to supine	I	S	Min	Mod	Max
WC Mobility - Propel on straight surfaces	I	S	Min	Mod	Max
Propel around comes & thru doors	I	S	Min	Mod	Max
Endurance for community	I		Min	Mod	Max
Transfers-Sit/stand & Stand/sit	I	S	Min	Mod	Max
WC/stand to low bed or toilet	I	S	Min	Mod	Max
WC/stand to floor	I	S	Min	Mod	Max
WC/stand to bathtub	I	S	Min	Mod	Max
WC/stand to car	I	S	Min	Mod	Max
Gait activities - Level surfaces	I	S	Min	Mod	Max
Ascends stairs	I	S	Min	Mod	Max
Descends stairs	I	S	Min	Mod	Max
Ramps	I	S	Min	Mod	Max
Endurance for community activities	I	S	Min	Mod	Max
ADL assessment - Bathing	I	S	Min	Mod	Max
Toileting	I	S	Min	Mod	Max
Dressing	I	S	Min	Mod	Max
Cooking	I	S	Min	Mod	Max

Conditions Requiring Special Precautions During Transfers

Conditions	Special Precautions
Total hip replacement, especially within first 2 weeks after surgery	■ Prevent hip adduction, internal rotation & flexion > 90° ■ No hip extension beyond neutral flexion-extension ■ Use a raised toilet seat & chair ■ Avoid excessive lumbar rotation, side & forward bend
Low back trauma or discomfort	■ Teach log rolling ■ Hips & knees should be partially flexed when in supine or side-lying

MS Diagnostics

Diagnostic Tests: X-ray

Indications: Initial test to evaluate what cannot be seen by observation; evaluate abnormalities from palpation

Info Gathered: Tumor, fracture, vascular abnormality, soft tissue abnormality, etc.

Precautions/Notes: Pregnancy

Diagnostic Tests: CT

Indications: To detect more info about any part of body

Info Gathered: Detailed visualization of parts scanned; location of tumors, tears, etc.

Precautions/Notes: Check for allergy to contrast (if contrast given); check if nervous in confined spaces

Diagnostic Tests: MRI

Indications: Detect changes in tissue not seen on CT or X-ray

Info Gathered: Changes in joints, ligaments, & cartilage; bone infection, disease, tumor, fracture; spine: disk herniation

Precautions/Notes: Check if claustrophobic; check on metal implants (those containing iron are contraindicated); check if contrast being used; pt may have allergy to contrast; check for pacemaker, artificial limbs, etc.; check if female has IUD

Diagnostic Tests: Radionuclide scintigraphy (bone scan)

Indications: Hot spot imaging to detect areas of fracture, NL or ABN bone healing, metastatic bone tumors, benign tumors, Paget's disease, AVN, osteomyelitis

Info Gathered: Reveals early bone disease or bone healing

Precautions/Notes: Not specific in differential diagnosis; must be used w/other lab, imaging, & clinical tests

Diagnostic Tests: Dual energy X-ray; absorptiometry

Indications: To evaluate bone mineral density: usually lower spine & hip areas evaluated

Info Gathered: Amount of Ca++ in certain regions of bones; estimation of bone strength; estimation of risk for fracture

Precautions/Notes: No known risks or side effects

Salter's Fracture Classification

Descriptors of Fracture	Definition
Site: Diaphyseal (a) Metaphyseal (b) Epiphyseal (c) Intra-articular (d)	(a) Shaft (b) Conical portion between shaft & epiphysis of long bone (c) Center of bone growth at articular end of bone (d) Within the joint
Extent: Complete or incomplete	If incomplete: can be crack, hairline, buckle, or green-stick fracture
Configuration: Transverse Oblique/spiral/comminuted	Complete fractures defined as crosswise across long axis (transverse), slanting (oblique), or spiral (coiled, winding around the long axis); more than 2 fragments (comminuted)
Relationship of fracture fragments: Displaced vs nondisplaced	If displaced: can be shifted sideways, angulated, rotated, distracted, overriding, or impacted

(Continued text on following page)

Salter's Fracture Classification (Continued)

Descriptors of Fracture	Definition
Relationship to external environment: Closed (simple) vs open (compound)	Closed: skin intact; Open: skin in area not intact
Complications: Complicated vs Uncomplicated	Complicated has either local or systemic complications; increases healing time

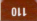

Types of fractures. (From Rothstein RM, Roy SH, Wolf SL: The Rehabilitation Specialist's Handbook, 3/e, p. 84.)

Special Considerations/Differential Diagnosis

Effect of Immobilization

Examples of Immobilization: Cast, Bedrest, Weightlessness, Denervation (SCI or Nerve Injury) Self-Imposed Due to Pain, Inflammation

Types of Tissue	Adaptation to ↓ Load	Result	Time for Change	Recovery
Ligament/ tendon	↓ Collagen content ↓ Cross-linking ↓ Tensile strength	Weakening of tissue	↓ tensile strength & stiffness by 50% after 8 wks	12–18 mo.
Articular surface (joint, menisci, underlying bone)	↓ Proteoglycan content ↓ Collagen synthesis Cartilage atrophy Regional osteoporosis ↓ Strength of ligaments at insertion sites ↑ H₂O content of cartilage	↓ ROM available to joint ↓ Time from load to failure ↓ Energy-absorbing capacity of bone-ligament complex Weakening of muscle around joint	Unknown	Unknown
Cartilage	Thinning of cartilage Advancing of subchondral bone	↓ ROM due to ↑ bone	Unknown	Unknown

(Continued text on following page)

Examples of Immobilization: Cast, Bedrest, Weightlessness, Denervation (SCI or Nerve Injury) Self-Imposed Due to Pain, Inflammation *(Continued)*

Types of Tissue	Adaptation to ↓ Load	Result	Time for Change	Recovery
Joint capsule	Disordered collagen fibrils AB cross-linking	Capsular stiffness, ↓ joint mobility	Unknown	Unknown
Synovium	Adhesion formation Fibro-fatty tissue proliferation into joint space	↓ Gliding, ↓ fluid movement	Unknown	Unknown
Muscle		Muscle atrophy: ■ Atrophy of type I fibers ■ If CNS damage: atrophy of type II fibers Joint contractures cause limits in ROM Alternate patterns of movement Vascular & fluid stasis	Within 3 days of immobilization	For every day of immobilization, may take up to 2 days of strengthening to return to NL strength

Fibromyalgia Screening

1. Do you have trouble sleeping through the night?	Yes	No
2. Do you feel rested in the morning?	Yes	No
3. Are you stiff & sore in the morning?	Yes	No
4. Do you have daytime fatigue/exhaustion?	Yes	No
5. Does your muscle pain & soreness travel to different places on your body?	Yes	No
6. Do you have tension/migraine headaches?	Yes	No
7. Do you have irritable bowel symptoms (nausea, diarrhea, cramping)?	Yes	No
8. Do you have swelling, numbness, or tingling in your arms/legs?	Yes	No
9. Are you sensitive to temperature & humidity or changes in the weather?	Yes	No

If yes to 2 or more questions, pt may have fibromyalgia.

Fibromyalgia tender points > 11 out of 18 is positive diagnosis.

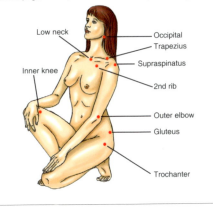

Low neck · Occipital · Trapezius · Supraspinatus · Inner knee · 2nd rib · Outer elbow · Gluteus · Trochanter

Osteoporosis Screening Evaluation

Evaluation Questions	Yes	No
1. Do you have a small, thin body?		
2. Are you white or Asian?		
3. Have any of your blood-related family members had osteoporosis?		
4. Are you a postmenopausal woman?		
5. Do you drink ≥ 2 oz of alcohol each day? (1 beer, 1 glass wine or 1 cocktail = 1 oz alcohol)		
6. Do you smoke more than 10 cigarettes each day?		
7. Are you physically active? (walk or similar exercise 3 ×/week)		
8. Have you had both ovaries removed before age 40 yr w/o hormone replacement?		
9. Have you been taking thyroid, anti-inflammatory, or seizure medications >6 mo?		
10. Have you broken your hip, spine, or wrist?		
11. Do you drink or eat >3 servings of caffeine, tea, coffee, or chocolate/day?		
12. Is your diet low in dairy products or other sources of calcium?		

If you answer yes to 3 or more questions, you may be at greater risk for developing osteoporosis

Evaluation of Incontinence

Types of Urinary Incontinence	Definition	Causes
Stress	Incontinence when ↑ pressure to bladder as in sneezing, laughing, exercising, coughing, heavy lifts	75% of all incontinence in women from stress: 1. Pelvic floor weakness 2. Ligament or fascia laxity 3. Urethral sphincter weakness Risk factors: pregnancy, vaginal delivery (long labor especially), heavy lifting, obesity, lack of hormone replacement in menopause, chronic constipation
Urge	Loss of urine when strong need to void (urgency)	1. Involuntary contraction of bladder 2. Involuntary sphincter relaxation 3. Alcohol, bladder infections, nerve damage, certain medications
Mixed (combination urge & stress)	Combination of pressure & strong urge	Muscle weakness plus involuntary contraction of bladder or involuntary sphincter relaxation
Overflow	Overdistention of the bladder	1. Acontractile bladder muscle 2. Hypotonic/underactive bladder muscle due to drugs, fecal impaction, diabetes, lower SCI, or disruption of motor nerve of bladder muscle (in MS)

(Continued text on following page)

Evaluation of Incontinence *(Continued)*

Types of Urinary Incontinence	Definition	Causes
		Men: mostly from prostate hyperplasia or carcinoma causing obstruction Women: severe genital prolapse or surgical overcorrection of urethral attachment causing obstruction
Bowel/bladder incontinence	Pressure or strong urge or gravity	Indication of SCI or nerve root damage

Comparison of Osteoarthritis & Rheumatoid Arthritis

Characteristics	OA	RA
Age of onset	Usually >40 yr	Usually >15 & <50 yr
Progression	Develops slowly over many yrs due to mechanical stress	May develop suddenly in wks/mos.
Manifestations	Osteophyte formation, cartilage destruction, altered joint alignment	Inflammatory synovitis, irreversible structural damage to joint & bone
Joint involvement	Few joints: DIP, PIP, first CMC of hands Cervical & lumbar spine Hips, knees, & first MTP of foot	Many joints, bilaterally MCP, PIP, hands, wrists, elbows, shoulders, cervical spine MTP, ankle

Comparison of Osteoarthritis & Rheumatoid Arthritis *(Cont'd)*

Characteristics	OA	RA
Joint signs/symptoms	Morning stiffness (>30 min) ↑ joint pain w/ weightbearing joints & activity	Redness, warmth, swelling, prolonged morning stiffness
Systemic signs/symptoms	Weightbearing joints Asymmetrical involvement	General feeling of sickness, fatigue Wt loss, fever, rheumatoid nodules Ocular, hematological, & cardiac symptoms Non–weightbearing joints Symmetrical involvement

Evaluation Notes for Practice Patterns

Preferred Practice Patterns for Musculoskeletal Conditions

Primary prevention/risk reduction for skeletal demineralization	Includes prolonged non-weightbearing; deconditioning, nutritional deficiency; menopause, hysterectomy, medications (e.g., steroids, thyroid medications, etc), chronic cardiovascular & pulmonary dysfunction
Impaired posture	Includes curvature of spine; disorders of back & neck; disk disorders; deformities of limbs; osteoporosis; muscle wasting, spasm; pregnancy-related problems, leg length discrepancy, joint stiffness
Impaired muscle performance	Includes pelvic floor dysfunction, chronic neuromuscular dysfunction, loss of muscle strength & endurance, arthritis, transient paralysis

(Continued text on following page)

Preferred Practice Patterns for Musculoskeletal Conditions (Continued)

Impaired joint mobility, motor function, muscle performance, & ROM associated w/*connective tissue dysfunction*	Includes joint subluxation or dislocation, ligament sprain, muscle sprain, prolonged immobilization, pain, swelling/effusion, arthritis, scleroderma, SLE
Impaired joint mobility, motor function, muscle performance, & ROM associated w/*localized inflammation*	Includes ankylosing spondylitis, bursitis, capsulitis, epicondylitis, fascitis, gout, OA, synovitis, tendonitis, muscle strain/weakness
Impaired joint mobility, motor function, muscle performance, ROM, & reflex integrity associated w/*spinal disorders*	Includes degenerative disk disease, spinal stenosis, spondylolisthesis, disk herniation, spinal surgery, ABN neural tension, altered sensation, muscle weakness, pain w/forward bending
Impaired muscle performance & ROM associated w/*fracture*	Includes bone demineralization & fracture, hormonal changes, medications, prolonged non-weightbearing state, muscle weakness from immobilization, trauma
Impaired joint mobility, motor function, muscle performance, & ROM associated w/*joint arthroplasty*	Includes arthroplastics, avascular necrosis, juvenile RA, neoplasms of the bone, OA, ankylosing spondylitis
Impaired joint mobility, motor function, muscle performance, & ROM associated w/*bony or soft tissue surgery*	Includes fusions, ankylosis, bone graft & lengthening, caesarean section, connective tissue repair, fascial releases, internal débridement, intervertebral disk disorder, laminectomies, muscle or ligament repair, open reduction internal fixation, osteotomies

Preferred Practice Patterns for Musculoskeletal Conditions *(Continued)*

Impaired joint mobility, motor function, muscle performance, ROM, gait, locomotion, & balance associated w/*amputation*	Includes amputation, frostbite, PVD, trauma

MS Interventions

More Common Orthotic, Protective, & Supportive Devices

Orthotic Defined by Location	Description/Indication
Cervical 1. Soft foam/rubber collar 2. Philadelphia collar 3. SOMI 4. Halo	1. Support the neck; ↓ work of neck muscles; minimal motion control 2. Rigid plastic supports chin & posterior head: greater motion control 3. Major restriction of all motion at neck w/four posts 4. Total restriction/maximal orthotic control: circular band of metal fixed to skull by four screws
Back 1. Lumbosacral orthosis (Knight spinal) 2. Thoracolumbosacral (Taylor brace)	1. Rigid trunk orthosis w/a pelvic & thoracic band & posterior uprights; restrains flexibility, controls extension, & limits lateral flexibility 2. Pelvic band & posterior uprights to midscapular level; reduces flexibility, lateral flexibility, & extension; limits trunk motion

(Continued text on following page)

More Common Orthotic, Protective, & Supportive Devices (Continued)

Orthotic Defined by Location	Description/Indication
Shoulder 1. Acromioclavicular separation splint 2. Hemiplegia sling	1. For management of an AC separation or postsurgery 2. Used post CVA to prevent trauma to AC joint & GH subluxation
Wrist 1. Static resting splints 2. Carpal tunnel splints	1. Maintains wrist joint in ext w/mild pressure to surface of hand; assists w/healing post surgery or post injury; may or may not splint each finger 2. Maintains wrist in neutral to prevent pressure on median nerve
Knee 1. Cho-Pat 2. Controlled motion knee brace 3. Palumbo patellar stabilization brace	1. Rubber strap placed at site of patellofemoral tendon 2. & 3. To protect area of injury, delimit extent of swelling & tissue damage, & control pt knee pain; also used to limit motion in sports activities for months after knee surgery
Ankle-Foot Orthosis	Plastic or metal orthoses used to compensate for paralysis of entire leg & provide dorsiflexion assistance; used in stroke, peripheral neuropathy, incomplete spinal cord injury

Muscle Fiber Types & Exercises to Increase Certain Muscle Fibers

Fiber Type	Common-Activity Muscles Most Active	Metabolic Capacity	Mitochondria	Exercises to → Fiber Recruitment
Fast twitch, type IIb	Stop & go, all-out exercise requiring rapid, powerful movements	Anaerobic	Absent	Short duration, ↑ speed, heavy lifting
Fast oxidative glycolytic, IIa	Fast-contracting, longer duration	Combination of aerobic & anaerobic	Present	Combination of ↑ speed or wt & ↑ duration
Slow twitch, type I	Slow speed of contraction, continuous activity	Aerobic	Present	Long duration, ↓ wt, multiple repetitions in strength ex.

MUS-

I. UE Diagonal Patterns

A. D1 flexion

Scapula-anterior elevation
Shoulder-flexion, adduction, ER
Elbow-varies
Forearm-supination
Wrist-radial flexion
Fingers-radial flexion
Thumb- flexion, adduction

B. D1 extension

Scapula-posterior depression
Shoulder-extension, abduction, IR
Elbow-varies
Forearm-pronation
Wrist-ulnar extension
Fingers-ulnar extension
Thumb- extension, abduction

C. D2 flexion

Scapula-posterior elevation
Shoulder-flexion, abduction, ER
Elbow-varies
Forearm-supination
Wrist-radial extension
Fingers-radial extension
Thumb- extension, abduction

D. D2 extension

Scapula-anterior depression
Shoulder-extension, adduction, IR
Elbow-varies
Forearm-pronation
Wrist-ulnar flexion
Fingers-ulnar flexion
Thumb- flexion, opposition

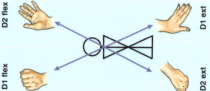

D1 flex   D2 flex

D2 ext   D1 ext

Neuroassessment

Cranial and Peripheral Nerve Integrity
Cranial Nerves: Functional Components

Number (Name)	Components	Function
I (Olfactory)	Afferent	Smell
II (Optic)	Afferent	Vision
III (Oculomotor)	Efferent (som)	Elevates eyelid, turns eye up, down, in
	VIs	Constricts pupil, accommodates lens
IV (Trochlear)	Efferent	Turns adducted eye down, causes eye twisting
V (Trigeminal)	Mixed: Afferent	Sensation from face, cornea, & anterior tongue
	Efferent	Mastication muscles, dampens sound
VI (Abducens)	Efferent	Turns eye out
VII (Facial)	Mixed: Afferent	Taste from anterior tongue
	Efferent (som)	Facial expression muscles Dampens sound
	Efferent (vis)	Tears/salivation
VIII (Vestibulo-cochlear)	Afferent	Balance (inner ear) Hearing
IX (Glosso-pharyngeal)	Mixed Afferent	Taste from posterior tongue Sensation from post-tongue, oropharynx
	Efferent	Salivation (parotid gland)
X (Vagus)	Mixed Afferent	Thoracic & abdominal viscera

(Continued text on following page)

Cranial Nerves: Functional Components (Continued)

Number (Name)	Components	Function
	Efferent	Larynx & pharynx muscles Decreases heart rate Increases GI motility
XI (Spinal Accessory)	Efferent	Head movements Sternocleidomastoid & trapezius
XII (Hypoglossal)	Efferent	Tongue movements & shape

Resisted Muscle Tests for Peripheral Nerve Integrity

Spinal Region Evaluated	Resisted Test for Dysfunction
C1	Cervical rotation force applied
C2, 3, 4	Shoulder elevation resisted
C5	Shoulder abduction resisted
C6	Elbow flexion at 90° resisted Wrist extension resisted
C7	Elbows flexed to 45°, elbow extension resisted Wrist flexion resisted
C8	Thumb extension resisted
T1	Fingers held in abduction resisted
L1, 2	Resisted hip flexion
L3, 4	Resisted dorsiflexion
L5	Great toe extension resisted
S1	Toe walk: 10-20 toe raises
S1, 2	Resisted knee flexion

If painful or painful and weak: muscular pathology
If painless and weak: neurological disorder

Neuromotor Development

Age	Gross Motor and Posture	Fine Motor	Cognitive
1 mo	Raises head while prone ABN reflexes present	Visual regard of objects Hands closed Swipes at objects	Scans within a face Shows preference for contrast
2 mo			Prefers NL face
3 mo	Rolls supine to side Rolls prone to supine accidentally	Glances from hand to object Reaches for but may not grasp object Visually directs reaching Hands clasped together often Sucking/swallow in sequence	
4 mo		Grasps rattle within 3 in Hands partially open	
5 mo	Rolls prone to supine segmentally	Holds objects	
6 mo	Supports self in sitting Begins to go to quadruped position	Thumb opposition; attempts to pick up objects Grasps and draws bottle to mouth	Imitates new behavior Searches for completely hidden object
7 mo	Crawls forward on belly Assumes quadruped position Begins pull to stand at furniture Begins getting to sit from prone	Reaches w/one hand while prone	Looks longer at scrambled face

(Continued text on following page)

Neuromotor Development ⚥ (Continued)

Age	Gross Motor and Posture	Fine Motor	Cognitive
8 mo	Reciprocal creep on all fours Cruises sideways at furniture	Reaches and grasps	
9 mo	Rises from supine by rolling to prone, pushing up to all fours	Feeds self crackers Holds bottle	
10 mo	Pulls to stand w/legs only Walks w/two hands held	Extends wrist, fingers Tries to feed self w/utensils	
11 mo	Takes independent steps Walking w/one hand held	Holds and drinks from cup Pincer grasp of finger foods	
12 mo	Walking		
13 mo		Crayon held w/fist	
14–16 mo	Walks up stairs while holding on		
17 mo	Walks down stairs while holding on		
18 mo			

Relationship Between Spinal Cord and Nerve Roots to Vertebral Bodies and Innervation of Major Muscle Groups

Physical Rehabilitation: Assess

	FUNCTIONAL LEVEL	MUSCLES PRESENT
Cervical nerves 1-8	C-1, C-2, C-3	– Facial Muscles
	C-4	– Diaphragm and Trap.
	C-5	– Deltoid and Biceps
	C-6	– Wrist Extensors
	C-7	– Triceps
	C-8, T-1	– Hand and Fingers
Thoracic nerves 1-12	T-2 – T-8	– Chest Muscles
	T-6 – T-12	– Chest Muscles
Lumbar nerves 1-5	L-1 – S-1	– Leg Muscles
Sacral nerves 1-5	S-1 – S-2	– Hip and Foot Muscles
	S-3	– Bowel and Bladder
Coccygeal nerve		

Reflex Integrity
Grading Scale for Muscle Stretch Reflexes

Grade	Evaluation	Response Characteristics
0	Absent	No muscle contraction w/reinforcement (palpable or visible)
1+	Hyporeflexic	Slight or slow muscle contraction; little to no joint movement. May require reinforcement to elicit contraction
2+	NL	Slight muscle contraction AND slight joint movement
3+	Hyperreflexia	Visible BRISK muscle contraction/moderate joint movement
4+	ABN	STRONG muscle contraction;1-3 beats of clonus
5+	ABN	STRONG muscle contraction w/sustained clonus

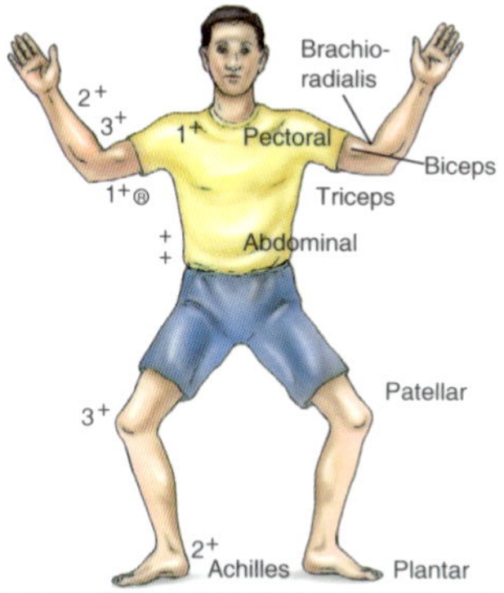

Brachio-radialis
2+
3+
1+ Pectoral
Biceps
1+ⓐ
Triceps
+
+ Abdominal
3+ Patellar
2+ Achilles
Plantar

Cutaneous Reflexes

Reflex	Description	NL Response	ABN Response
Abdominal	Scratching of skin of anterior abdominal wall w/sharp object (*lateral to medial scratch* in a single dermatome) Evaluates integrity of T6-L1	Deviation of umbilicus toward stimulus	May be absent in obese pt or late pregnancy Loss of reflex; corticospinal (pyramidal) system disease Loss on one side; stroke
Cremasteric	Stroking of skin of proximal & medial aspect of thigh; involves L1, L2	Elevation of testicle in response to stroking	No response in injury to lumbosacral segments of spinal cord or lesions in pyramidal system
Bulboca-vernous	Pinching of glans penis; involves S2-S4	Palpable contraction of bulbospongiosus meatus at base of penis	Lack of response w/injury to conus medullaris or sacral spinal roots
Anal Sphincter	Scratching of perianal skin; involves S2-S4	Contraction of external anal sphincter	Lack of response w/injury to conus medullaris & complete SCI above L2
Plantar (most commonly tested)	Stimulus to sole of foot in sweeping motion: calcaneus → distally over shaft of 5th metatarsal, → medially metatarsal heads; stimulus: even pressure for 1 sec; knee: fully extended (L5-S2)	Plantar flexion of toes produced by contraction of flexor digitorum longus, flexor hallucis longus, & lumbrical muscles of foot	Babinski's response: dorsiflexion of great toe and fanning of lateral four toes; found in corticospinal damage

ABN Muscle Stretch Reflexes: Present in UMN or Frontal Lobe Damage

ABN Reflexes	Description
Jaw (cranial nerve V)	Depression of jaw slightly w/finger; percuss finger to open jaw further + reflex: jaw closes reflexively
Snout (cranial nerve VII)	Percussion of upper lip at midline in philtrum region + reflex: puckering or pursing of lips
Glabellar (cranial nerve VII)	Percussion of glabella of eye + reflex: blinking when tapped
Hoffmann's (median nerves C6–C8)	Flick distal phalanx of long finger: wrist in neutral & metacarpophalangeal joint in slight extension + reflex: when thumb & index finger move toward opposition

Modified Ashworth Scale for Grading Spasticity

Grade	Description
0	No increase in muscle tone
1	Slight ↑ in tone; catch and release OR minimum resistance at end of ROM when moved in flexion or extension
1+	Slight ↑ in tone; catch followed by minimum resistance throughout ROM
2	Moderate ↑ in tone through most ROM but body parts move easily
3	Considerable ↑ in tone; passive movement difficult
4	Affected part(s) rigid in flexion or extension

Tone Definitions

Abnormalities	Types	Definitions
Spasticity: velocity-dependent ≠ in tone	Clasp: knife reflex	Passive stretch produces high resistance, followed by sudden letting go
	Clonus	Cyclical, spasmodic hyperactivity of antagonistic muscles; common in calf muscles
	Decerebrate rigidity	Sustained contraction & posturing of trunk & limbs in **full extension**; exaggerated spasticity
	Decorticate rigidity	Sustained contraction & posturing of trunk & **lower limbs** in extension & upper limbs in flexion; exaggerated form of spasticity
Rigidity: resistance uniformly ↑ in both agonist & antagonist muscles; body parts stiff and immoveable	Cogwheel rigidity	Rachet-like response to passive movement = alternate letting go & ↑ resistance to movement
	Lead pipe rigidity	Constant rigidity
Flaccidity (hypotonia): ↓ or absent muscle tone		Resistance to passive movement diminished; stretch reflexes are ↓; limbs are floppy; joints may hyperextend Weak or paralysis: can be temporary (spinal shock) from UMN or CVA or long-lasting from LMN
Dystonia: hyperkinetic movement disorder: impaired or disordered tone, sustained involuntary movements		Tone fluctuates unpredictably from low to high; dystonic posturing: sustained twisting deformity Seen in central deficit: inherited or w/neurodegenerative disorders or metabolic disorders; also seen in spasmodic torticollis (wry neck)

Reflex Testing in Pediatric Patients

	Reflex	Stimulus	Response
Primitive/ spinal	Flexor Withdrawal	Pinprick to sole of foot in supine or sit position	Toes extend, foot dorsiflexes, leg flexes Integrated 1-2 mo
	Crossed Extension	Noxious stimulus to ball of foot while extremity in extension; pt supine	Opposite LE flexes, then adducts and extends Integrated 1-2 mo
	Traction	Grasp forearm, pull up from supine to sit	Total flexion of UE Onset 28 wk gestation Integrated 2-5 mo
	Moro	Sudden change in position of head	Extension, abduction of UE Integrated 5-6 mo
	Startle	Sudden loud noise	Extension or abduction of arms Persists through life
	Grasp	Pressure to palm of hand or ball of foot	Flexion of fingers or toes Integrated 4-6 mo; fingers, 9 most toes
Tonic/Brain Stem	Asymmetrical tonic neck	Rotation of head to one side	Fencing posture Integrated 4-6 mo

MUS

Reflex Testing in Pediatric Patients (Continued)

Reflex	Stimulus	Response
Symmetrical tonic neck	Flexion or extension of head	Flexion of head causes arm flexion, leg extension With head extension: arm extension, leg flexion Integrated 8–12 mo
Symmetrical tonic labyrinthine	Prone or supine position	Prone: ↑ flexor tone Supine: ↑ extensor tone Integrated 6 mo
Positive supporting	Pressure on ball of foot in stand position	Rigid extension of LE Integrated 6 mo
Associated reactions	Resisted voluntary movement in any part of body	Involuntary movement in resting extremity Integrated 8–9 yr
Neck righting action on the body	Passively turn head to one side while pt supine	Body rotation as a whole (log roll) Integrated 5 yr
Body righting acting on the body	Passively rotate upper or lower trunk segment	Body aligns w/rotated segment Integrated 5 yr
Labyrinthine head righting	Occlude vision, tip body in all positions	Head orients to vertical position Persists

(Continued text on following page)

Reflex Testing in Pediatric Patients (Continued)

Reflex	Stimulus	Response
Optical righting	Alter body position by tipping in all directions	Head orients to vertical position Persists throughout life
Body righting acting on head	Place prone or supine	Head orients to vertical Integrated 5 yr
Protective extension	Displace center of gravity outside base of support	Arms/legs extend and abduct to support & protect Persists
Equilibrium reactions: tilting	Displace center of gravity by tilting or moving the support surface	Trunk curves toward upward side; extension & abduction of extremities on side; protective extension on opposite Persists
Equilibrium reactions: postural fixation	Apply displacing force to body; alter center of gravity	Trunk curves toward external force w/extension & abduction of extremities on side force was applied Persists

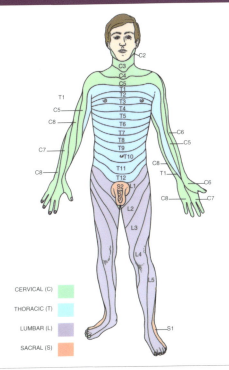

CERVICAL (C)

THORACIC (T)

LUMBAR (L)

SACRAL (S)

Sensory Testing (Continued)

	Method of Testing	Response
Pain: sharp/dull	Use pin & dull object (use sharp & dull parts of same pin): ask "without look-ing, tell if object is sharp or dull"	↑ When crossed spinothalamic tract cut (e.g.: for chronic pain)
Temperature	Use hot & cold tap water in tube: "tell if object feels warm or cold"	Identifies dysfunction in anterolateral pathways
Light touch	Dab cotton ball on skin; ask when and where touched	↓: Look for anatomic pattern for nerve injury; ABN in multiple nerve & root areas: brain/ brainstem lesion ↑ In all extremities: periph-eral polyneuropathy + Loss of motor: spinal cord injury
Position sense	Passive joint (fingers, toes, wrist, or ankle) displacement	↓: Dysfunction of joint or muscle receptors, disease in large myelinat-ed primary afferents, or sensory processing center dysfunction
Vibration	After tapping tuning fork to set it, apply fork handle to bony prominences & nails	↑: Peripheral nerve disease affecting large fibers (demyelinated neuro-pathy) or in central demyelination; shows functional recovery of demyelinated nerve fibers

Sensory Testing *(Continued)*

	Method of Testing	Response
Stereognosis	Pt asked to identify common objects placed in hand	↓ w/Lesion of multiple ascending pathways or parietal lobe
Two-point discrimination	Determines spatial localization; compass w/blunted tips applied w/↓ distances between tips until one tip reported	Crude measure of discriminative sensation
Bilateral simultaneous stimulation	With subject's eyes closed, lightly touch one side, then other side of body; pt determines which side & where	Parietal lobe disease: feel stimulus on one side only
Graphesthesis	Tracing letters or numbers w/finger on palmar surface of hand	↓ w/Damage to dorsal columns, medial lemniscus, ventral post thalamus, or parietal lobe

Two-point discrimination

From Gulick D, OrthoNotes, Philadelphia, F.A. Davis Co., 2005, p. 118.

Classification of Clinical Tests of Sensory Function

Functional System	Clinical Tests
Anterolateral systems	Pin prick, thermal sense Deep pain
Dorsal column: medial lemniscus	Light touch, vibratory sense Position sense
Cortical sensory function	Traced figure identification Object identification, double simultaneous stimulation

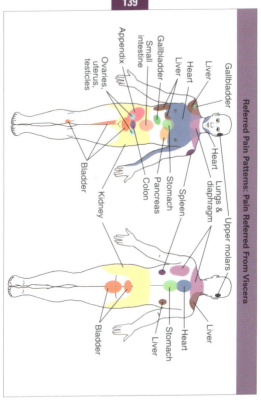

Referred Pain Patterns: Pain Referred From Viscera

Gallbladder
Liver
Heart
Liver
Gallbladder
Small intestine
Appendix
Ovaries, uterus, testicles
Bladder
Kidney
Colon
Pancreas
Stomach
Heart
Spleen
Lungs & diaphragm
Upper molars
Heart
Bladder
Stomach
Liver
Heart
Liver

Assessment of Thoracic Outlet Syndrome

Testing for proximal compression of subclavian artery, vein, and/or brachial plexus involves placing pt in several positions that may provoke compression of these structures.

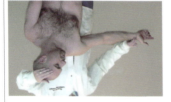

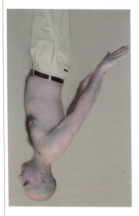

Test: Examiner monitors radial pulse of affected extremity

Response: Pulse rate slows: + test for compression of subclavian artery by anterior scalene muscle

Test: Retract & depress shoulders from relaxed position: exaggerated military position

Response: Onset of symptoms or radial pulse slowing indicates + test for compression of neurovascular bundle

Assessment of Thoracic Outlet Syndrome *(Continued)*

Test: Move affected arm(s) into abduction position: monitor pulse & symptoms
Response: Onset of symptoms or radial pulse slowing

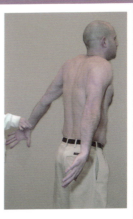

Test: 3-min elevated arm test: arms abducted to 90° & elbows flexed to 90°; alternately, open & close hands
Response: + if unable to complete 3 min or onset of symptoms

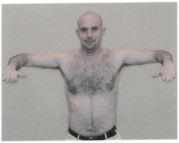

Balance Assessment
Balance Tests and Responses

Components	Balance Responses	Tests	
Sensory elements	Detects orientation of body & body parts in reference to environment Includes: ■ Visual system ■ Somatosensory system ■ Vestibular system	Assess of vertigo Automatic postural reaction Crossed extensor tests Cutaneous function Flexor withdrawal Postural muscle activity Angular & linear acceleration & deceleration forces on head Righting reactions of head, trunk, limbs Visual acuity w/Snellen Eye Chart	Proprioception Regulation of muscle tone Stabilization of gaze Stretch reflex tests Visually guided movements Visual field tests
Sensory interaction	Sense of equilibrium: sense of position of center of mass in relation to support surface	Assess stand balance w/different sensory conditions ■ Surfaces: dense foam/NL/other ■ Visual input varies from eyes closed to open	
Musculoskeletal elements	Simple stretch reflex to functional stretch reflex to postural synergies and equilibrium reactions	ROM Tone Evaluate posture (static balance) & movement (dynamic) & response to balance disturbance Assess for postural synergies	Strength

Functional Balance Tests

Test	Description
Berg Balance Scale	Evaluates posture/control w/14 conditions: w/↓ base of support in sit/stand/single leg stance
Functional Reach Test	Evaluates ability to reach forward w/o feet moving
Timed Up and Go	Evaluates dynamic balance/mobility: timed activity of rise from chair, stand, walk 3 M, return & sit
Balance measures: parallel, semi-tandem, tandem stand	Length of time to maintain balance during different foot positions

Functional Balance Grades

Grade	Description
NL	Able to maintain balance w/o support Accepts max challenge & shifts wt
Good	Able to maintain balance w/o support Accepts mod challenge & shifts wt but some limitations evident
Fair	Able to maintain balance w/o support Cannot tolerate challenge; cannot maintain balance w/wt shift
Poor	Requires support to maintain balance
Zero	Requires max assist to maintain balance

Memory Tests
Mental Status Tests

Elements Tested	Description	Examples of Tests
Level of consciousness	Alert Stupor Lethargic Coma Obtunded	Observation by fam
Attention	Ability to focus and remain w/o distraction on a stimulus or task	Ask about medical hx, recite months backwards, recite a list of digits provided
Orientation	Person Place Time	What is your name? Where are you? What day/year is it? Who is the current president?
Language function	Fluency Repetition Comprehension Spontaneous speech Naming and word finding	Questions on personal events, word problems, fam, common interests
Reading and writing	Learning and memory Immediate recall Short-term Long-term	Recall of distant news events, word problems, math problems
Cortical and cognitive functions	Fund of knowledge Ability to perform calculations Proverb interpretation Praxia/ apraxia Gnosia/agnosia	Calculations Recall of messages Proverbs
Mood and affect	Feelings, emotions, & soma-tic & autonomic behaviors: determine if appropriate in current situation	Observation
Thought content	Fullness & organization of thinking: (paranoia: disor-dered thought content)	Stories, personal experiences, & fam hx questions

Coordination Tests

Test	Description	Abnormalities
Alternate heel to knee or toe	Supine: touch knee & big toe alternately w/heel of opposite extremity	Cerebellar dysfunction: slow/dysrhythmic
Alternate nose to finger	Sitting: touch tip of nose & tip of therapist's finger w/index finger; change position of therapist's finger	Cerebellar dysfunction: ataxic, slow
Draw a circle	Pt draws imaginary circle in air w/upper or lower extremity; may be performed supine	Cerebellar disease: ataxic, slow
Finger to finger	Shoulders abducted to 90° w/elbows extended; pt brings both index fingers to midline & touches fingers	Slow w/intention tremors
Finger to nose	Shoulders abducted to 90° w/elbows extended; pt brings tip of index finger to tip of nose	Cerebellar disease: unsteady or shaky movements; action or intention tremors
Finger opposition	Tip of thumb pressed to tip of each finger in sequence; ↑ speed gradually	Dysdiadochokinesia: inability to perform rapid contraction/relaxation
Finger to therapist's finger	Sitting opposite, therapist holds finger in front of pt who is required to touch finger as therapist moves finger around	Slow or dysrhythmic

(Continued text on following page)

Coordination Tests (Continued)

Test	Description	Abnormalities
Rebound test	Elbow flex: therapist applies manual resistance to produce isometric contraction of biceps: resistance suddenly released	Opposing muscle group (triceps) does not contract and "check" movement
Pronation/ Supination	Elbows flexed to 90° & held close to body. Pt alternately turns palms up and down ↓ Speed gradually	Slow or dysrhythmic
Tapping foot	Taps ball of foot on floor w/o raising knee; heel keeps contact w/floor	Slow movement, unable to hold heel on floor
Tapping hand	With elbow flexed, forearm pronated, pt taps hand on knee	Slow movement, unable to perform rapid tapping
Fixation or hold position	UE: pt holds arms horizontally in front. LE: pt holds knee in extended position	Unable to hold arms or knees in position; ataxic movements

Tests for Autonomic Function

HR/BP	Signs of Postural Hypotension
Bowel/ bladder	Incontinence Reflexive emptying of bowel/bladder
Signs of sympathetic hyperactivity	Excessive sweating Palpitations Elevated BP Flushing Tachycardia Nasal stuffiness Arrhythmias Pounding headache Pale or mottled skin appearance Goose bumps (piloerection)
Signs of sympathetic dystrophy (reflex sympathetic dystrophy)	Trophic changes: ■ Change in skin & nail texture/skin color ■ Loss of hair Edema Lack of sweating Poor peripheral temperature regulation
Observe for Horner's syndrome	Miosis (papillary dilation) Ptosis (partial drooping of eyelid) Anhydrosis (lack of sweating) Flushing of face
Observe difficulties w/swallowing	Hoarseness
Observe for GI disturbances	Nausea, vomiting, changes in GI motility

Upper vs Lower Motoneuron Lesions: Signs and Symptoms

Signs/Symptoms	UMN	LMN
Paresis/plegia	Spastic	Flaccid
Deep tendon reflexes	Increased	Decreased or absent
Passive stretch response	Velocity-sensitive increase in resistance	↓ Compliance of muscles
Ability to isolate muscle contractions	Loss of ability to isolate muscle contractions	Retention of ability to isolate muscle contractions
Muscle strength	Inappropriate stereo-typic movement patterns w/ volitional movement; muscle strength difficult to determine	Atrophy of affected muscles
EMG results	Increased activity	EMG evidence of denervation
Babinski's & Hoffman's signs	Positive	Negative

Spinal Cord Injury Bowel & Bladder Changes

Dysfunction	Bowel	Bladder	Sexual Functioning
Spinal shock	No reflexive movement	Flaccid: no tone	No reflexes seen
UMN	Reflex bowel: responds to digital stimulation	Contract/reflex empty in response to level of filling pressure Reflex arc intact Intermittent catheterization usually used	M: Reflexogenic erectile function (only 3% ejaculate) Reflexogenic sexual arousal (lubrication, engorgement, clitoral erection) F: Fertility/pregnancy unimpaired, often early labor
LMN	Autonomous/nonreflex bowel: relies on straining & manual evacuation	Nonreflex bladder: flaccid Emptied by ↑ intra-abdominal pressure/ Crede's maneuver & timed voiding	M: Often no erections 25% psychogenic erections 15% ejaculate F: No reflex sexual arousal: + psychogenic responses Fertility/pregnancy unimpaired, often early labor
Incomplete	Usually similar to complete UMN	Usually similar to complete UMN	M: 98% reflexogenic erectile function F: Reflexogenic sexual arousal

Glasgow Coma Scale

Eye Opening	Pts	Best Verbal Response	Pts	Best Motor Response	Pts
Spontaneous: indicates arousal mechanism in brainstem is active	4	Oriented: knows person, place, time	5	Obeys commands (no involuntary movements)	6
To sound: eyes open to sound stimuli	3	Confused: responds to questions w/some disorientation or confusion	4	Localized: moves a limb to attempt to remove stimulus	5
To pain: apply stimulus to limbs, not face	2	Inappropriate: speech understood; unable to sustain conversation	3	Flexor: NL Entire shoulder or arm is flexed in response to painful stimulus	4
Never opens eye	1	Incomprehensible: unintelligent sounds such as moans, groans	2	Flexion: ABN Assumes decorticate rigidity posture w/painful stimuli	3
		None	1	Extension: ABN adduction & internal rotation of shoulder; pronation of forearm	2
				None	1

Rancho Los Amigos Cognitive Function Scale

Score	Scale Description
X	Purposeful & appropriate: handles multiple tasks simultaneously in all environs/may require breaks Independently initiates assistive memory devices
IX	Purposeful & appropriate: independently shifts back & forth between tasks, completes accurately for 2 hr Uses assistive memory devices
VIII	Purposeful & appropriate: recalls past & recent events & aware of environment Shows carry-over for new learning
VII	Automatic - appropriate: appears appropriately & oriented in hospital & home settings/robot-like
VI	Confused - appropriate: depends on external input or direction/follows simple directions
V	Confused - inappropriate: responds to simple commands consistently/responses not appropriate w/↑ complexity & lack of external structure
IV	Confused-agitated: heightened state of activity/bizarre behavior/nonpurposeful
III	Localized response: reacts specifically but inconsistently to stimuli
II	Generalized response: reacts inconsistently & nonpurposefully to stimuli in nonspecific way
I	No response

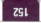

Common Causes of Unconsciousness

Condition	Manifestation
Acute alcoholism	Stuporous; responds to noxious stimuli; alcoholic breath; eyes moderately dilated; equal reactive pupils; respirations deep and noisy; blood alcohol >200 mg/dL
Cranial trauma	Often local evidence or hx of injury; pupils unequal and sluggish or inactive; pulse variable; BP variable; reflexes altered; may have incontinence and paralysis; CT reveals intracranial hemorrhage or fracture
Stroke: ischemia or hemorrhage	Usually hx of CVD or hypertension; sudden onset w/asymmetry; pupils unequal and inactive; focal neurological signs; hemiplegia
Epilepsy	Sudden convulsive onset; may have incontinence; pupils reactive; tongue bitten or scarred
Diabetic acidosis	Onset gradual; skin dry, face flushed; fruity breath odor; hyperventilation, ketonuria, hyperglycemia, metabolic acidosis in blood
Hypoglycemia	Onset may be acute w/convulsions; preceded by lightheadedness, sweating, nausea, cold/clammy skin, palpitations, headache, hunger; Hypothermia, pupils reactive, deep reflexes exaggerated, + Babinski's sign
Syncope	Onset sudden, associated w/emotional crisis or heart block; coma seldom deep or prolonged; pallor; slow pulse rapid & weak; Awakens promptly when supine
Drugs	Cause of 70% of acute coma w/unknown cause

Neurodiagnostics

Diagnostic tests/Indications	Information From Tests	Precautions/Notes
Clinical EMG: needle insertion for single motor unit potentials; to study motor unit activity & integrity of neuromuscular system; identifies denervated areas of muscle and myopathic changes	Records electrical activity present in contracting muscle Identifies LMN disorders & nerve root compression & distinguishes neurogenic from myopathic disorders	Examiner judges pt effort, determines if recruit is NL Inaccurate placement: distorts recorded potentials Interpretation problems w/ anatomical anomalies: accuracy improves w/experience in interpretation
Kinesiological EMG: to examine muscle function during specific purposeful tasks	Patterns of muscle response, onset & cessation of activity & level of response Used to facilitate or inhibit specific muscle activity	Compare information gathered from nerve conduction velocity Same precautions as clinical EMG
Nerve conduction velocity: uses surface electrodes; to assess peripheral nerves: sensory and motor	Evaluation of peripheral neuropathies, motoneuron disease, demyelinating disorders	Routine testing does not pick up peripheral neuropathy affecting small unmyelinated C fibers Early peripheral neuropathy may show absent sensory but NL motor

(Continued text on following page)

Neurodiagnostics (Continued)

Diagnostic tests/Indications	Information From Tests	Precautions/Notes
EEG; to assess any brain dysfunction, especially epilepsy	Differential Dx of seizures: especially if spontaneous attack; no EEG activity: Dx of brain death	Sensitive but not specific; inexpensive
Magnetoencephalography; to assess any brain dysfunction: epilepsy	NEW: records magnetic field produced by brain's electrical activity	Better than EEG
CT scan; to identify structural diseases of brain & spinal cord	Diagnostic test of choice for evaluation of disease of brain/spine associated w/acute trauma, intra- or subarachnoid hemorrhage, bony lesions of skull, cervical/lumbar root lesions, & brachial or lumbosacral plexus lesions	Expensive; cannot diagnose metabolic or inflammatory disorders Used instead of MRI in presence of metal, including pacemaker or cerebral aneurysm clips; or if pt agitated or claustrophobic

Neurodiagnostics (Continued)

Diagnostic tests/Indications	Information From Tests	Precautions/Notes
Lumbar puncture: to confirm suspicion of CNS infection; before anticoagulant therapy for cerebrovascular disease	Cell count & differential Cytological exam for neoplastic cells Stains for bacteria & fungi Culture for organisms	Contraindicated if tissue infection in region of puncture site Complications of test: headache & backache
Angiography: to visualize blood vessels of brain & spinal cord	Evaluate cerebrovascular disease, cerebral venous sinuses, intracranial aneurysms & spinal A-V anomalies	Evaluate pt for contrast dye allergies

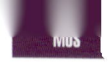

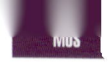

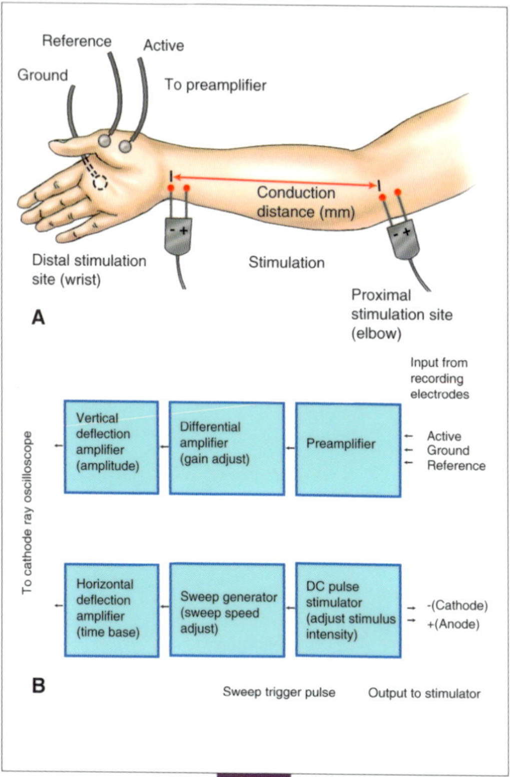

A

Reference Active
Ground
To preamplifier

Distal stimulation
site (wrist)

Conduction
distance (mm)

Stimulation

Proximal
stimulation site
(elbow)

B

To cathode ray oscilloscope

Vertical deflection amplifier (amplitude)	Differential amplifier (gain adjust)	Preamplifier

Input from recording electrodes
— Active
— Ground
— Reference

Horizontal deflection amplifier (time base)	Sweep generator (sweep speed adjust)	DC pulse stimulator (adjust stimulus intensity)

→ –(Cathode)
→ +(Anode)

Sweep trigger pulse   Output to stimulator

Quick Screen

Motor control assessment: all areas should be checked as ABN vs NL

NL	ABN	Test
___	___	Cognition
___	___	Communication
___	___	Arousal
___	___	Sensation
___	___	Perception
___	___	Flexibility
___	___	Tone
___	___	Deep tendon reflexes
___	___	Developmental reflexes
___	___	Righting reactions
___	___	Muscle strength
___	___	Movement patterns
___	___	Coordination
___	___	Balance
___	___	Gait
___	___	Functional abilities

Neuromuscular Interventions

Procedural Interventions	Specific Activities
Balance, coordination, & agility training	Developmental activities training
	Motor control and learning training/retraining
	Neuromuscular education/re-education
	Perceptual training
	Postural awareness training
	Sensory training/retraining
	Task-specific performance training
	Vestibular training

(Continued text on following page)

NEURO-

Neuromuscular Interventions *(Continued)*

Procedural Interventions	Specific Activities
Body mechanics and postural stabilization	Body mechanics training
	Postural control training
	Postural stabilization activities
	Posture awareness training
Gait and locomotion training	Developmental activities training
	Gait training
	Perceptual training
	Wheelchair training
Neuromotor development training	Motor training
	Movement pattern training
Flexibility exercises	Muscle lengthening & stretching; ROM exercises
Strength, power, & endurance training	Active assistive, active resistive exercises (concentric/eccentric, isokinetic, isometric, isotonic) Task-specific performance training
Electrotherapeutic modalities	Biofeedback
	Electrical stimulation
Physical agents and mechanical modalities	Pulsed electromagnetic fields Cryotherapy Hydrotherapy Light: infrared/laser/ultraviolet Sound: phonophoresis/ultrasound Thermotherapy: diathermy/dry heat/hot packs/paraffin Compression therapies: bandaging/ garments/taping/contact casting/ vasopneumatic compression Gravity-assisted compression devices: stand/tilt table CPM traction devices: intermittent/ positional/sustained

Neuromuscular Interventions *(Continued)*

Procedural Interventions	Specific Activities
Functional training in self-care and home management	ADL training Barrier accommodations/ modifications Device/equipment use & training Functional training programs: back school, simulated environments, task adaptation, travel training IADL training Injury prevention or reduction
Functional training in work, community, and leisure	Same as self-care and home management but in work, community, or leisure setting

Special Considerations/Populations

Potential Problems w/Spinal Cord Injury

Problem	Symptoms	Description
Autonomic Dysreflexia	Hypertension Bradycardia Profuse sweating ↑ Spasticity Headache Vasodilation above lesion Goose bumps	**Pathological reflex in lesions above T-6; episodes ↓ over time; rare after 3 yr postinjury** Acute onset from noxious stimuli below level of injury: bladder distention, rectal distention, pressure sores, urinary stones, bladder infection, noxious cutaneous stimuli, kidney malfunction, environmental temperature changes Treat medical emergency: assess catheter for kinks; change position; assess source of irritation: bladder irrigation or bowel

(Continued text on following page)

NEURO

Potential Problems w/Spinal Cord Injury (Continued)

Problem	Symptoms	Description
Postural Hypotension	↑ in BP w/ change in position to upright	Loss of sympathetic vasoconstriction control associated w/lack of muscle tone, < in cervical & upper thoracic lesions. Develop edema in legs, ankles, & feet. Treatment: Adapt to vertical position slowly, compress stockings & abdominal binder, meds to ↑ BP diuretics to ↑ edema
Heterotopic Bone Formation	Loss of ROM	Osteogenesis (bone formation) in soft tissues below level of lesion: Problems w/joint motion & function extracapsular and extra-articular Treatment: drugs; physical therapy for ROM; surgery
Contractures	Severe limitations in ROM	Develops secondary to position: prolonged shortening Causes: lack of active muscle, gravity, positioning
DVT	Local swelling, erythema, & heat	Thrombus (clot) develops in vein; may travel to lungs: ↑ risk of pulmonary embolus & cardiac arrest Treatment: anticoagulation (heparin first)
Osteoporosis Renal calculi	Stone formation Fracture, postural changes	Net loss of bone mass: ↓ risk for fracture: ↑ estimated risk first 6 mo; postinjury ↓ Ca++ in blood, ↑ risk of stone formation
Pressure sores	Erythema, skin breakdown	Ulcerations of soft tissue: from pressure (wt); see Tab 5

Communication Disorders

Disorder	Description
Aphasia Anomic	Difficulty naming objects; word-finding problems
Broca's	Difficulty expressing mild difficulty understanding complex syntax
Conduction	Difficulty in repetition of spoken language; word-finding pauses & letter or whole word substitutions
Crossed	Transient; occurs in RH persons w/R hemisphere lesion; ↓ comprehension
Global	Most common & severe form; spontaneous speech: few stereotypical words/sounds; comprehension ↓ or absent; repetition, reading, & writing: impaired
Subcortical (thalamic)	Dysarthria & mild anomia w/ comprehension deficits; in lesions of thalamus, putamen, caudate, or int cap
Transcortical	Spontaneous speech restricted: able to repeat, comprehend, & read well
Wernecke's	Severe disturbance in auditory comprehension w/inappropriate responses to questions
Agraphia	Writing ability disturbed; associated w/aphasia; found in lesions in post-language area or frontal language area
Aprosody	Disturbance of melodic qualities of language; change in intonation patterns or expressive language
Dysarthria	Result from loss of control of muscles of articulation

American Spinal Injury Association Classification

Impairment Scale	Description
A: Complete transaction of spinal cord	No motor or sensory function is preserved in the sacral segments S4-S5
B: Incomplete	Sensory but not motor is preserved below neurological level
C: Incomplete	Motor function preserved below neurological level: > than half of key muscles below neurological level have < grade 3
D: Incomplete	Motor function preserved below neurological level, at least half of key muscles below neurological level have a muscle grade = or >3
E: NL	Motor and sensory function are NL

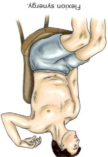

Flexion synergy.

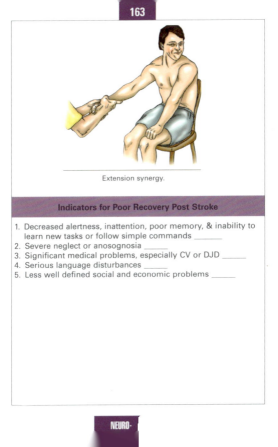

Extension synergy.

Indicators for Poor Recovery Post Stroke

1. Decreased alertness, inattention, poor memory, & inability to learn new tasks or follow simple commands _____
2. Severe neglect or anosognosia _____
3. Significant medical problems, especially CV or DJD _____
4. Serious language disturbances _____
5. Less well defined social and economic problems _____

Synergy Patterns in Stroke

	Flexion Synergy Components	Extension Synergy Components
Upper extremity	Scapular retraction/ elevation or hyperextension	Scapular protraction
	Shoulder abduction/ external rotation	Shoulder adduction*/internal rotation
	Elbow flexion*	Elbow extension
	Forearm supination	Forearm pronation*
	Wrist & finger flexion	Wrist & finger flexion
Lower extremity	Hip flexion,* abduction, external rotation	Hip extension, adduction*, internal rotation
	Knee flexion	Knee extension*
	Ankle dorsiflexion, inversion	Ankle plantar flexion*, inversion
	Toe dorsiflexion	Toe plantar flexion
*Strongest component		

Guide to PT Practice: Preferred Practice Patterns for Neuromuscular

Preferred Practice Pattern: Primary prevention/risk reduction for loss of balance and falling

Includes: Advanced age, alteration to senses, dementia, depression, dizziness, hx of falls, meds, musculoskeletal diseases, neuromuscular diseases, prolonged inactivity, vestibular pathology

Preferred Practice Pattern: Impaired neuromotor development

Includes: Alteration in senses, birth trauma, cognitive delay, genetic syndromes, developmental coordination disorder, developmental delay, dyspraxia, fetal alcohol syndrome, prematurity

Preferred Practice Pattern: Impaired motor function & sensory integrity associated w/nonprogressive CNS disorders: congenital origin or acquired in infancy or childhood

Includes: Brain anoxia/hypoxia, birth trauma, brain anomalies, cerebral palsy, encephalitis, premature birth, traumatic brain injury, genetic syndromes (w/CNS), hydrocephalus, infectious disease (w/CNS), meningocele, neoplasm, tethered cord

Preferred Practice Pattern: Impaired motor function & sensory integrity associated w/nonprogressive CNS disorders acquired in adolescence or adulthood

Includes: Aneurysm, brain anoxia/hypoxia, bell's palsy, CVA, infectious disease (affects CNS), intracranial neurosurgical procedure, neoplasm, seizures, traumatic brain injury

Preferred Practice Pattern: Impaired motor function & sensory integrity associated w/progressive CNS disorders

(Continued text on following page)

NEURO-

Guide to PT Practice: Preferred Practice Patterns for Neuromuscular (Continued)

Includes: AIDS, alcoholic ataxia, Alzheimer's diseases, ALS, basal ganglia disease, cerebellar ataxia, cerebellar disease, idiopathic progressive cortical disease, intracranial neurosurgical procedures, Huntington's disease, multiple sclerosis, neoplasm, Parkinson's disease, primary lateral palsy, progressive muscular atrophy, seizures

Preferred Practice Pattern: Impaired peripheral nerve integrity & muscle performance associated w/peripheral nerve injury

Includes: Neuropathies: carpal or cubital tunnel syndrome's palsy, radial or tarsal tunnel syndrome; peripheral nerve disorders: labyrinthitis, paroxysmal positional vertigo; surgical nerve lesions, traumatic nerve lesions

Preferred Practice Pattern: Impaired motor function & sensory integrity associated w/acute or chronic polyneuropathies

Includes: Amputation, Guillian-Barré syndrome, postpolio syndrome, axonal polyneuropathies: alcoholic, diabetic, renal, ANS dysfunction, leprosy

Preferred Practice Pattern: Impaired motor function, peripheral nerve integrity, & sensory integrity associated w/nonprogressive disorders of the spinal cord

Includes: Benign spinal neoplasm, complete/incomplete spinal cord lesions, infectious diseases of spinal cord, spinal cord compression: degenerative spinal joint disease, herniated disk, osteomyelitis, spondylosis

Preferred Practice Pattern: Impaired arousal, range of motion, & motor control associated w/coma, near coma, or vegetative state

Includes: Brain anoxia, birth trauma, CVA, infectious/ inflammatory disease affecting CNS, neoplasm, premature birth, traumatic brain injury

APTA: Guide to Physical Therapist Practice, 2nd ed. Physical Therapy, 2001;81:9-744.

Assessment

Assessment of integumentary system includes:

- Activities, positioning, & postures that produce or relieve trauma to skin (observations, pressure-sensing maps, scales)
- Assistive, adaptive, orthotic, protective, supportive equipment that may produce or relieve trauma to skin
- Skin characteristics include:
  - Blistering
  - Continuity of skin color
  - Dermatitis
  - Hair growth
  - Mobility
  - Nail growth
  - Sensation
  - Temperature
  - Texture
  - Turgor
- Burn description & quantification
- Wound characteristics:
  - Bleeding
  - Contraction
  - Depth
  - Drainage
  - Exposed anatomical structures
  - Location
  - Odor
  - Pigment
  - Shape
  - Size
  - Staging, progression, & etiology
  - Tunneling
  - Undermining
  - Pulses/vascular tests
  - Periwound: girth, edema, etc.
  - Pain
- Wound scar tissue characteristics:
  - Banding
  - Pliability
  - Sensation
  - Texture
- Signs of infection
  - Cultures
  - Observations
  - Palpation

Classification of Burn Injury

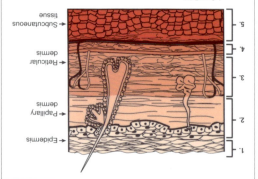

1. Superficial
2. Superficial partial thickness
3. Deep partial thickness
4. Full thickness
5. Subdermal

Epidermis →
Papillary dermis →
Reticular dermis →
Subcutaneous tissue →

Classification of Burn Injury (Continued)

Classification	Characteristics			Appearance	Healing
	Sensation	Blisters	Color		
Superficial	Pain/ tenderness delayed	Usually absent	Red	Dry, but edema may be present	Healing occurs w/o scarring
Superficial partial thickness	SEVERE	Intact blisters	Red	Bubbled w/blisters, edema	Minimal or no scarring
Deep partial thickness	Painful, but less severe than superficial	Broken	Mixed red or waxy white	Moderate edema/WET from broken blisters	Healing occurs w/hypertrophic scars & keloids
Full thickness	Anesthetic to pain & temp	None	White, brown, black, or red	Hard, parchment-like eschar formation or leathery, dry	Infection common Grafts necessary/ skin regenerates only from edges of burn
Subdermal	Anesthetic	None	White, brown, black, or red	Necrotic tissue throughout	Extensive surgery necessary to remove necrotic tissue; may need to amputate

Types of Burn Injuries

Type	Cause	Wound Characteristics
Thermal burn	Skin exposed to flame	Wounds have irregular borders Depth of injury varies
	Sudden explosion or ignition of gases: flash burns	Exposed surfaces burned uniformly Usually result in partial-thickness burns
	Hot objects (metals): contact burns	Deep, sharply circumscribed wounds All skin elements & underlying structures destroyed
Scald burns	Contact w/hot liquids	Superficial wounds Hot liquid remains in contact w/skin for time (immersion/clothing holding liquid in contact), deep-partial or full-thickness injuries result
Chemical	From acids or strong alkalies	Tissue may be exposed for long periods unless washed immediately Result in partial- or full-thickness damage
Electrical	Electrical current	Cause well-circumscribed, deep injuries involving muscle, tendon, bone Neurovascular structures involved Injuries result in severe movement dysfunction & physical disability

Extent of Burned Area:
Rule of Nines for Estimating Burn Area

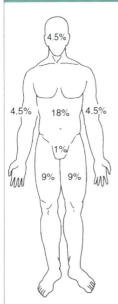
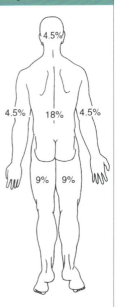

Adults. (From Rothstein JM, Roy SH, Wolf SL. The Rehabilitation Specialist's Handbook, 3/e. 2005.)

Extent of Burned Area:
Rule of Nines for Estimating Burn Area (Continued)

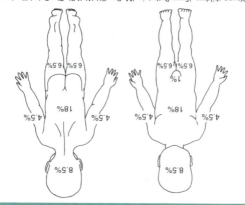

Young children. (From Rothstein JM, Roy SH, Wolf SL. The Rehabilitation Specialist's Handbook, 3/e. 2005.)

Secondary Complications of Burn Injury

2° Comp	Description	Signs/Symptoms
Infection	Inflammation phase: ↑ risk of mortality; wound at risk due to ↑ edema, ↓ defense, & ↑ resistance to antibiotic Burns: systemic & topical antibiotics Wounds: topical antibiotics	Fever, lethargic, ↓ WBC Bacterial count >10⁶ means wound infection; >10⁷ associated w/↑ risk of mortality

Secondary Complications of Burn Injury *(Continued)*

2° Comp	Description	Signs/Symptoms
Pulmonary	Suspect inhalation injury w/burn in a closed space (incidence >33%) or facial burns; ↑ risk of mortality Complications: CO poisoning, tracheal damage, upper airway obstruction, pulmonary edema, pneumonia; later complications: restrictive disease, inhalation injury, late sequelae (advanced restrictive disease) Perform xenon lung scan & serial PFT	Facial burns, singed nasal hairs, harsh cough, hoarseness, ABN breath sounds, respiration distress, sputum w/carbon, hypoxemia
Metabolic	Rapid ↓ body wt, negative nitrogen balance, ↓ energy stores, change in glucose kinetics in result in hyperglycemia Treat w/nutrition, ↓ room temperature	↑ Core temperature, ↓ body wt, ↑ sweat & heat loss in room at NL temperature; ↓ albumin, globulin, protein; ↑ free fatty acids, triglycerides
Cardiac function/circulatory	Significant ↓ plasma & intravascular fluid volume; initial ↓ cardiac output (may ↓ 30% within first 30 min), alterations in platelet concentration & function, RBC dysfunction	↓ RBC, ↑ HR

Secondary Complications of Burn Injury (Continued)

2° Comp	Description	Signs/Symptoms
Musculoskeletal	Significant damage to bone or peripheral circulation may result in amputation; significant ↓ wt results in loss of muscle mass & fiber atrophy	↑ Sarcomeres; ↑ ROM; muscle atrophy, osteoporosis, heterotopic ossification (pain, sudden loss of ROM within 3-12 wk after injury)
Neurological	Often seen in electrical injuries; involves spinal cord, brain, & peripheral nerves; often peripheral neuropathies; scar tissue formation may also cause nerve compression	Peripheral neuropathies, ↓ sensation, ↑ edema, ↓ strength
Pain	Pain limits spontaneous movement & exercise; when wound open: pain ↑, when wound closed: pain ↑; lubrication critical to avoid pain & skin cracking	Itching, ↓ sensitivity to heat, cold, touch

Burn Wound Healing

Area of Healing	Phase	Description
Dermal	Inflammatory	Begins time of injury; ends 3-5 days; leukocytes ↓ contamination; redness, edema, warmth, pain, ↓ ROM
	Proliferative	Surface: re-epithelial; deep: fibroblasts (cells synthesize scar tissue) migrate & proliferate; collagen deposited w/random alignment; stresses (stretching): fibers align along path of stress Granulation tissue formed (macrophages, fibroblasts, & blood vessels) Wound contraction occurs; skin grafts may ↓ contracture
	Maturation	Remodeling of scar: 2 yr/↓ in fibroblasts, vasculitis ↓, collagen remodels, & ↑ strength; hypertrophic scar: red, raised, firm; rate of collagen production > rate of collagen breakdown Keloid: large, firm scar/overflows wound boundaries
Epidermal		Surface of wound: cells migrate & cover wound; damage to sebaceous glands may cause dryness & itching during healing; external lubrication needed

INTEG

Classification of Ulcers

Etiology	Location	Defining Characteristics
Vascular ulcers: arterial	Distal lower extremities	Location: toes, feet, shin; Pain: severe unless neuropathy masking pain; Gangrene: may be present; Signs: ↓ pulses, trophic changes, cyanosis when dependent
Vascular ulcers: venous insufficiency	Distal lower extremities	Pain: not severe; Surrounding skin: pigmented, fibrotic; Gangrene: absent; Signs: edema, stasis dermatitis. Location: inner or outer ankle. Tracing to assess wound size.
Trophic ulcers (decubitus or pressure sores); usually due to impaired sensation	Over bony prominences	Location: in areas w/diminished sensation; usually secondary to immobilization; Surrounding skin: callous; Pain: absent; Signs: ↓ sensation, ↓ ankle jerks
Diabetic foot ulcers	Distal position, around toes, deep into foot	Extremely aggressive & may lead to serious complications such as amputations; ↑ risk of infection

Risk Factors for Pressure Ulcers

Risk Factor	Preventive Actions	
Bed/chair confinement	Inspect skin 1 x/day; bathe daily, prevent dry skin Avoid use of doughnut-shaped cushions; participate in rehabilitation program ↓ friction on skin by lifting (do not drag) & corn starch on skin	
	Bed confinement	Chair confinement
	Change position q 2 hr	Change position q 1 hr
	Use foam, air, gel, H_2O mattress	Use foam, gel, or air cushion to relieve pressure
Inability to move	Reposition q hr Change position q 15 min if can not shift wt in chair Use pillows/wedges to keep knees & ankles from touching Place pillow under midcalf in bed to keep heels from touching	
Loss of bowel or bladder control	Clean skin whenever soiled/assess & treat urine leaks If constant moisture: use absorbent pads w/quick-drying surface Protect skin w/cream or ointment	
Poor nutrition	Eat balanced diet/consider nutritional supplement	
Lowered mental awareness	Choose preventive actions that apply If confined to bed or chair, change position as noted above	

Other Risk Factors in Wound Care

Circulation: poor circulation increases risk
Chemotherapy: overall cell destruction
Steroid therapy: ↓ inflammatory response
Presence of systemic infection
Diabetes: ↓ circulation & sensation
Repeated trauma: ↑ friction injury
↓ Age: ↓ epithelial turnover & elasticity
↑ Albumin &/or ↓ prealbumin: malnutrition

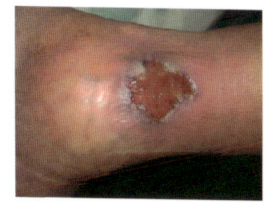

Venous ulcer. (Courtesy of Dr. Benjamin Barankin.)

Stages & Etiology of Pressure Wounds
(from AHCPR classification guidelines)

Stage	Description	Etiology: out→in	Etiology: inside→out
I	Redness (discoloration in pigment skin) w/o breakdown & will not blanch; warm, edema, induration, or hardness	Pressure to skin distorts superficial blood vessels: ischemia & leakage	Pressure on deep muscle decreases blood flow to skin
II	Partial-thickness skin loss (epidermis, dermis, or both), abrasion, blister/shallow crater	Prolonged superficial pressure leads to more necrosis	Pressure on perforators is extensive, leading to ↓ blood flow to skin
III	Full-thickness skin loss, damage or necrosis to subcutaneous tissue, may extend to underlying fascia; presents as deep crater with or w/o undermining tissue	Persistent external pressure	Distortion of deep blood vessels by pressure of bone or muscle impairs blood flow
IV	Full-thickness skin loss with increased tissue necrosis/damage to muscle w/exposed bone or supporting tissues; undermining	Extremely high pressure & prolonged: affects deep blood vessels	Prolonged pressure on blood vessels is severe; muscle necrosis

Wound Characteristics From Wound Bed Assessment

Characteristics	Indications	Diagnostic Technique	Concerns/Additional Comments
Color	Look for signs of clinical infection Evaluate progress of therapeutic regimen	Photos & color coding: look at black, yellow, red areas; analyze color by computer software; w/o software, use pictures	Maintain standard protocol: Same camera Same lighting Same distance from wound Same flash on camera
Odor	Assessment of bacteria	Electronic noses Clinical: description of odor	Electronic nose $$$; not found in clinic Description of odor doesn't tell specific bacteria involved
Temperature	↑ Temperature associated w/infection ↓ Temperature slows healing;↓ O_2 release Chronic leg wounds: 24-26°C	Infrared thermography Glass mercury thermometers or electronic display devices using thermistors	Expensive/not widely available in clinic Thermometers: More easily understood & more widely used
pH	Intact skin: 4.8-6.0, Interstitial fluid = neutral pH monitors healing: acidification from chemicals increases healing	Flat glass electrode	Wound pH measurement used to predict skin graft survival, wound healing under synthetic dressings, etc
Area & volume	Defines progress of healing	3D mapping from scanned images; clinical use of photos/tracings of wound & depth measures	Recorded at baseline & weekly intervals

Special Considerations/Populations

Identifying Skin Cancers

Cancers	Etiology	Warning Signs
Malignant melanoma: one of most virulent cancers Courtesy of Dr. Benjamin Barankin.	Excessive exposure to sun Heredity Atypical moles	Change in surface of a mole: Scaliness/oozing/ bleeding Spread of pigment from border → surrounding skin Change in sensation (itchiness, tenderness, pain)
Basal cell carcinoma Courtesy of Dr. Benjamin Barankin.	Most common cancer in whites Risk factors: light hair, eyes, com- plexions; tan poorly	Fleshy bump or nodule on head, neck, or hands: rarely metasta- sizes but can extend below skin

(Continued text on following page)

Identifying Skin Cancers *(Continued)*		
Cancers	**Etiology**	**Warning Signs**
Squamous cell carcinoma	Second most common skin cancer found in whites Develops into large masses: can me-tastasize	Appear as nodules or red, scaly patches; found on rim of ear, face, lips, & mouth

Other Skin Problems

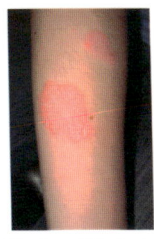

Psoriasis. (Courtesy of Dr. Benjamin Barankin.)

Etiology: Genetic/noncontagious; appears as a result of a "trigger": Emotional stress, injury to skin, drug reaction, some infections

Warning Signs: Generalized fatigue, tenderness/swelling, or pain over tendons, morning stiffness, redness & rash, swollen fingers/toes

Interventions

Topical Meds Frequently Used in Burn Treatment

Med	Description	Application
Polysporin (bacitracin)	Clear ointment; used for gram-positive infections	Small amount applied directly to wound: keep uncovered
Accuzyme (collagenase)	Enzymatic débriding (necrotic tissue selectively); no antibacterial effects	Apply to eschar, cover w/moist dressing with or without antibacterial agent
Furacin (nitrofurazone)	Antibacterial cream for less severe burns; ↓ bacterial growth	Applied directly on wound or gauze dressing
Gentamycin	Antibiotic for gram-negative, staph & strep bacteria	Applied w/sterile glove; covered w/gauze
Silver sulfadiazine	Most commonly used antibacterial agent; used especially for *Pseudomonas*	White cream applied w/sterile glove 2-4 mm thick to wound or into mesh gauze; may be left open
Sulfamylon (mafenide acetate)	Topical antibacterial; used for gram-negative or -positive; diffuses through eschar	White cream applied directly to wound (1-2 mm thick) 2 x/day; left open or w/thin layer of gauze
Silver nitrate	Antiseptic germicide & cleanser; penetrates only 1-2 mm eschar; for surface bacteria; stains black	Used every 2 hr in dressings or soaks; also available in small sticks

INTEG

INTEG

Wound Dressings/Treatments*

Type of Dressing	Brand Name	Clinical Tips
Thin films (polyurethane films)	Opsite Tegaderm Polyskin Bioclusive	For stage I, II w/minimal drainage, NO infection Nonabsorbent, permeable to gas, contraindicated on fragile skin, works well w/moist dressings, works over joints
Hydrocolloid	Comfeel Plus Ulcer dressing Comfeel Plus Transparent Dressing Granuflex Bordered DuoDerm Extra Thin Tegasorb	For stage I, II, III w/minimal to moderate drainage & NO infection Aggressive adhesion, not effective in dry wounds Difficult to visualize surrounding skin Moderately absorbent Not indicated in stage IV
Alginate/CMC fibrou dressing	SeaSorb Soft Dressing Aquacel dressing Sorbsan dressing	For stage II, III, IV w/moderate to excessive wound drainage Absorbs exudates, maintains wound moisture, semipermeable, requires 2nd dressing, requires careful removal

184

Wound Dressings/Treatments* *(Continued)*

Type of Dressing	Brand Name	Clinical Tips
Hydrogels	Purilon gel IntraSite gel Duoderm Hydroactive gel Solosite Vigilon	For stage II, III, IV, & nonstageable w/minimal drainage, NO infection Assists in débridement by hydration; nonadherent; difficult to keep in place ↓ pain, closes naturally; requires a secondary dressing, semipermeable
Foam dressings	Blatain Non-adhesive Blatain Adhesive Allevyn Non-adhesive Allevyn Adhesive Mepilex Mepilex border	For stage III, IV w/excessive drainage & NO infection Nonadherent, absorbs large amount exudates; semipermeable
Absorptive dressings (granular exudates absorbers)	Bard Absorption dressing Hydragan Debrisan	For stage III, IV w/wound drainage, NO infection Good filler for deep wounds, keeps moist, used to débride w/ autolysis Difficult to keep in place, requires 2nd dressing, semipermeable

*Wound dressings are constantly revised & newer ones may be available

INTEG

Skin Grafts & Flaps Used in Burn Treatment

Skin Graft/Flap	Description
Advancement flap	Local flap: skin next to wound moved to cover defect w/detachment from original site
Allograft (homograft, cadaver)	Graft taken from donor but not genetically identical to recipient
Autograft	Graft taken from recipient's body
Delayed graft	Graft partially elevated & replaced: moved to another site
Free flap	Skin tissue moved to a distant site where vascular reconnection is made
Full-thickness graft	Graft that contains all layers of skin but no subcutaneous fat
Heterograft	Graft taken from member of another species
Isologous	Graft from donor who is genetically identical to recipient
Local flap	Relocation of skin to adjacent site w/part of flap remaining attached to its own blood supply
Mesh graft	Donor's skin cut to form mesh: expanded to cover a larger area
Myocutaneous flap	Flap w/muscle, subcutaneous fat, skin, & patent blood supply
Pedicle flap	Flap w/one end attached: allows blood supply to reconnect new end
Rotational flap/ Z-plasty	Local flap: section incised on three sides & pivoted: covers area next to it
Sheet graft	Donor skin applied w/o alteration to recipient's damaged area
Split-thickness graft	Graft w/only superficial dermal layers

Positioning for Common Deformities

Joint	Common Deformity	Motions to be Stressed	Approaches to Positioning
Neck: anterior	Flexion	Hyperextension	Position neck in extension or use rigid cervical orthosis
Shoulder/axilla	Adduction/internal rotation	Abduction, flexion, External rotation	Position w/shoulder flexed & abducted
Elbow	Flexion/pronation	Extension/supination	Splint in extension
Hand	Claw hand (intrinsic minus)	Wrist extension, MCP flexion, proximal & distal ICP extension, thumb palmar abduction	Wrap fingers individually, elevate for edema; use intrinsic positive, wrist in extension, MCP flexion, proximal & distal ICP in extension, thumb in palmar abduction w/web space
Hip/groin	Flexion/adduction	All motions, especially hip extension, abduction	Hip neutral, extension w/slight abduction
Knee	Flexion	Extension	Posterior knee splint
Ankle	Plantar flexion	All motions	Plastic ankle-foot orthosis, ankle positioned in 0° dorsiflexion

(Continued text on following page)

INTEG

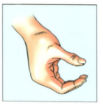

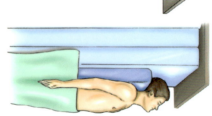

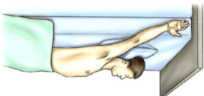

Positioning for Common Deformities (Continued)

Electrotherapy Treatments for Burns/Wounds

Modality	Indication
Infrared	Fungal infections, psoriatic lesions
Hydrotherapy	Cleanse & enhance wound healing
Electric stimulation	To enhance wound healing

Adjunctive Interventions in Wound Healing

Intervention: Normothermia

Description: Delivery of warm moist heat from infrared heating element inserted into dressing; treatment: three 1-hr treatments/d

Contraindications: Cannot be used on third-degree burns

Intervention: UV radiation therapy

Description: UV lamp plus commercial product: derma wand or Handisol; use UV depending on desired treatment effect

Contraindications: TB, systemic diseases (renal, liver, cardiac, or lupus), cancer in wound, fever, acute psoriasis, herpes simplex or eczema

Intervention: Negative pressure therapy

Description: Apply controlled level of subatmospheric pressure (50-125 mm Hg < ambient pressure) to interior of wound; open cell polyurethane foam dressing, apply via pump in continuous vacuum

Contraindications: None.

Intervention: Hyperbaric O_2 therapy

Description: Pt breathes OR tissue is surrounded by 100% O_2 at pressures > NL atmospheric pressure (O_2 delivery 2-3x > atmospheric pressure); indications: gas gangrene, problem wounds, necrotizing soft tissue infection, osteomyelitis, thermal burns, crush injuries

(Continued text on following page)

Adjunctive Interventions in Wound Healing (Continued)

Contraindications: Toxic effects if used improperly: S/s of O_2 toxicity: dry cough, nausea/vomiting, pulmonary fibrosis, visual changes, seizures; contraindications: seizure disorders, malignant tumor

Intervention: Platelet-derived growth factor
Description: Topically applied bioengineered growth factor to accelerate healing; particularly for diabetic foot ulcer
Contraindications: Limited evidence of efficacy on wounds except diabetic foot

Intervention: Stem cell therapy
Description: Pluripotential stem cells differentiate into fibroblasts, endothelial cells, & keratinocytes
Contraindications: Found in bone marrow: currently controversy exists w/use of stem cells

Practice Patterns of Integumentary Disorders

Practice Patterns	Includes Individuals With
Primary prevention/risk reduction for integumentary disorders	Amputation, CHF, diabetes, malnutrition, neuromuscular dysfunction, obesity, peripheral nerve involve, polyneuropathy, prior scar, SCI, surgery, vascular disease
Impaired integumentary integrity associated w/superficial skin involvement	Amputation, burns (superficial & first-degree), cellulitis, contusion, dermopathy, dermatitis, malnutrition, neuropathic ulcers (grade 0), pressure ulcers (grade 2), vascular disease (arterial, diabetic, venous)
Impaired integumentary integrity associated w/ partial-thickness skin involvement & scar formation	Amputation, burns, derm disorders, epidermolysis bullosa, hematoma, immature scar, malnutrition, neoplasm, neuropathic ulcer, pressure ulcer, prior scar, d/s post SCI, surgical wounds, toxic epidermal necrolysis, traumatic injury, vascular ulcers

Practice Patterns of Integumentary Disorders *(Continued)*

Practice Patterns	Includes Individuals With
Impaired integumentary integrity associated w/full-thickness skin involvement & scar formation	Amputation, burns, frostbite, hematoma, scar (immature, hypertrophic, or keloid), lymphostatic ulcer, malnutrition, neoplasm, neuropathic ulcers, pressure ulcers, surgical wounds, toxic epidermal necrolysis, vascular ulcers
Impaired integumentary integrity associated w/skin involvement extending into fascia, muscle, or bone & scar formation	Abscess, burns, chronic surgical wounds, electric burns, frostbite, hematoma, Kaposi's sarcoma, lymphostatic ulcer, necrotizing fasciitis, neoplasm, neuropathic ulcers (grades 3, 4, 5), pressure ulcers (stage 4), recent amputation, subcutaneous arterial ulcer, surgical wounds, vascular ulcers

APTA: Guide to Physical Therapist Practice, 2nd ed. Physical Therapy 2001;81:9-744.

LABS

General Chemistry

Lab/Normal Values	Deviations & Causes
Albumin/3.5–5.0 g/ 100 mL	↓ in chronic liver disease; protein malnutrition, malabsorption syndrome, chronic infection, acute stress
Aldolase/1.3–8.2 U/L	↑ in muscle or bone damage or disease
Alkaline phospha-tase/13–39 U/L infants-adolescents >104 U/L	↑ in liver & bone diseases (obstructive & hepatocellular liver disease), obstructive jaundice, biliary cirrhosis, etc. ↓ in osteomalacia, metastatic bone disease & slightly ↑ in healing fractures
Ammonia/ 2–55 μmol/L	↑ in hepatic encephalopathy & Reye's syndrome; tested to evaluate changes in consciousness
Amylase/4–25 U/mL	↑ in acute pancreatitis (first hrs, NL in 2–3 days); ↓ for weeks/months w/chronic pancreatitis; ↑ in peritonitis, perforated peptic ulcer, acute intestinal obstruction, mesenteric thrombosis, & inflammation of salivary glands (e.g. mumps)
Anion gap/ 8–16 mEq/L	A calculated value using the results of electrolyte panel ↓ w/metabolic acidosis (e.g., uncontrolled diabetes, starvation, kidney damage, intake of toxic substances), ↑ aspirin, methanol) ↑ w/l albumin or w/l immunoglobulins
AST, SGOT/8–46 U/L (M); 7–34 U/L (F)	↓ in heart, liver, & skeletal muscle diseases ↑ in acute MI, necrosis of heart muscle (myocarditis); acute liver damage, cirrhosis, metastatic CA, obstructive jaundice, infectious mono, congestive hepatomegaly; ↑ in muscle disease: gangrene of muscle, dermatomyositis, crush injury, & ingestion of aspirin, codeine, & cortisone

General Chemistry (Continued)

Lab/Normal Values	Deviations & Causes
Bilirubin total/ <1.0 mg/100 mL	↑ w/destruction of RBCs: hemolytic diseases, hemorrhage, hepatic dysfunction, transfusion-initiated hemolysis, autoimmune disease
BNP/<100 pg/mL	↑ w/heart failure <500 goal for hospital D/C >700 decompensated heart failure
BUN/8-25 mg/100 mL	↑ w/high protein intake, dehydration, burns, GI hemorrhage, renal disease, prostate hypertrophy ↓ w/↓ protein ingestion, starvation, liver dysfunction, cirrhosis
Calcitonin/0-14 pg/mL 0-28 pg/mL	↑ in C-cell hyperplasia & MTC; used to screen: risk for MEN 2
Calcium/8.5-10.5 mg/100 mL	↑ w/↑ vitamin D intake, osteoporosis, ↓ Na, ↓ urinary excretion, immobilization, ↑ Ca reabsorption, hypothyroidism ↓ w/↓ vitamin D intake, pregnancy, excessive diuretic, starvation ↓ $Mg++$, acute pancreatitis, hypoalbuminemia
Carbon dioxide content/bicarbonate or CO_2/24-30 mEq/L	Altered w/electrolyte imbalance; chronic disease, especially kidney disease; & to evaluate acid-base balance; ↑ indicates alkalotic compensation or disease, ↓ in acidic compensation or metabolic acidosis
Chloride	↓ w/$K+$-sparing diuretics, vomiting, excess ingestion of $K+$ ↑ (rarely) w/diarrhea, NH_4Cl ingestion
Cholesterol/<200 mg/dL	↑ indicates ↑ risk for heart disease
Cortisol/5-25 μg/100 mL (before noon) <10 μg/ 100 mL (after noon)	↓ in Addison's disease & anterior pituitary hypofunction; ↑ Cushing's syndrome & stress

(Continued text on following page)

General Chemistry (Continued)

Lab/Normal Values	Deviations & Causes
Creatine/0.2-0.5 mg/dL (M); 0.3-0.9 mg/dL (F)	↓ in kidney disease/monitoring of progression of kidney function
Creatine kinase/ 17-148 U/L (M); 10-79 U/L (F)	↓ in heart or skeletal muscle, progressive muscular dystrophy, cerebral infarcts ↑ isoenzymes distinguish origin of CPK (MM↑: skeletal muscle injury; MB↑: cardiac muscle; BB↑: brain injury)
Creatinine/0.6-1.5 mg/100 mL	↓ in renal disease/renal failure, chronic glomerulonephritis, hyperthyroidism
Ferritin/10-410 ng/dL	↑ in chronic iron deficiency or if proteins are severely depleted, malnutrition ↓ in chronic iron excess (hemochromatosis)
Folate/2.0-9.0 ng/mL	↑ in vegan vegetarians & malnutrition, malabsorption as in celiac disease, Crohn's disease, & cystic fibrosis; ↑ in pernicious anemia, ↑ stomach acid production, bacterial overgrowth in stomach, liver & kidney disease, alcoholism
Glucose/70-110 mg/100 mL	↓ in diabetes, pancreatic insufficiency, steroid use, pancreatic neoplasm, thiazide diuretics, excess catecholamines ↑ in beta cell neoplasm, hypothyroidism, starvation, glycogen storage diseases, Addison's disease
Iron/50-150 µg/100 mL	↑ in anemia (as in chronic bleeding from gut or ↓ loss from heavy menstrual periods), chronic diseases such as cancers, autoimmune diseases, & chronic infections ↓ in hemochromatosis, excessive iron ingestion, & heavy alcohol ingestion

General Chemistry *(Continued)*	
Lab/Normal Values	**Deviations & Causes**
Iron binding capacity or transferring/250-410 μg/ 100 mL	↑ in iron-deficiency anemia ↓ w/hemochromatosis, anemia from chronic infection or chronic disease, in liver disease (cirrhosis), & when ↓ protein in diet & in nephritic syndrome
Lactic acid (lactate)/ 0.6-1.8 mEq/L	↑ in hemorrhage, shock, sepsis, DKA, strenuous exercise, cirrhosis
Lactic dehydrogenase/45-90 U/L Has 5 isoenzymes	LDH1 ↑: MI, myocarditis, anemia, shock, malignancy LDH2 ↑: MI, myocarditis, anemia, chronic granulocytic leukemia, pulmonary infarction, shock, malignancy LDH3 ↑: leukemia, pulmonary infarction, mononucleosis, shock, malignancy LDH4 ↑: mononucleosis, shock, malignancy LDH5 ↑: CHF, hepatitis, cirrhosis, skeletal muscle necrosis dermatomyositis, mononucleosis, shock, malignancy
Lipase/<2 U/mL	↑ in pancreatitis (very high) & kidney disease, salivary gland inflammation, & peptic ulcer; may be ↑ briefly w/tumor
Magnesium/1.5-2.0 mEq/L	↑ w/↑ Ingestion of Mg++ (antacids) ↓ Malabsorption syndrome, acute pancreatitis
Osmolality/280-296 mOsm/kg H₂O	↑ w/dehydration ↓ w/fluid overload
Phosphorus/ 3.0-4.5 mg/100 mL	↑ w/↑ Growth hormone, chronic glomerulonephritis, sarcoidosis ↓ in hyperinsulinism, ↓ ingestion phosphorus
Potassium/ 3.5-5.0 mEq/L	↓ w/excess diuretic use, vomiting, cirrhosis, licorice intake, fasting/starvation ↑ in kidney disease, trauma, burns, excess replacement

(Continued text on following page)

General Chemistry (Continued)

Lab/Normal Values	Deviations & Causes
Prealbumin/ 18-32 mg/dL	↓ Poor nutrition/malnutrition Used to monitor nutrition w/parenteral nutrition
Prostate-specific antigen/0-4.0 ng/mL	A tumor marker to screen for prostate cancer; ↑ in prostate cancer, prostatitis, & benign prostatic hyperplasia
Protein – total/ 6.0-8.4 g/100 mL	This information is not helpful unless know albumin & globulin levels.↑ or ↓ in kidney disorder or when protein not absorbed; estrogen & oral contraceptives also ↑ protein
Sodium/135-145 mEq/L	↑ in dehydration (burns, sweating, diarrhea), diuretics H_2O retention (CHF renal, cirrhosis, excess intake), renal dysfunction, excess IV therapy ↓ w/excess H_2O loss, poor H_2O intake, hyperaldosteronism
T3/75-195 ng/100 mL	↑ hypothyroidism, rare pituitary hyperthyroidism ↓ hypothyroidism
T4 free/ 0.75-2.0 ng/dL	More accurate reflection of thyroid ↑ hypothyroidism, rare pituitary hyperthyroidism ↓ hypothyroidism
T4 total/4-12 µg/ 100 mL	Original test for thyroid function; now replaced w/free T4 ↓ in hypothyroidism, ↑ in hyperthyroidism
Thyroglobulin/ 3-42 µ/mL	Functions as tumor marker to assess effectiveness of thyroid cancer treatment & monitor recurrence; ↑ may indicate recurrence

General Chemistry *(Continued)*

Lab/Normal Values	Deviations & Causes
Triglycerides/ 40-150 mg/100 mL	↑ in CAD, diabetes, nephritic syndrome, hepatic disease, & hypothyroidism
TSH/0.5-5.0 µ/mL	↑ indicates underactive thyroid, pituitary tumor, or lack of response to thyroid meds; ↓ indicates overactive thyroid or too much response to meds
Urea nitrogen/ 8-25 mg/100 mL	↑ in impaired kidney function from acute/chronic kidney disease or ↓ blood flow to kidneys (CHF, shock, MI, burns); also ↑ in excess protein breakdown or ↑ dietary protein or excess bleeding; ↓ liver disease, malnutrition, & overhydration
Uric acid/ 3.0-7.0 mg/100 mL	↑ in chronic lymphocytic & granulocytic leukemia, multiple myeloma, chronic renal failure, fasting, including ingestion of protein; gout, fasting, toxemia in pregnancy, ↑ salicylate ingestion, excess alcohol intake

Rehabilitation Implications of General Chemistry

Abnormal Lab Test Result	Implications for Rehabilitation
↓ Albumin	If malnourished, may have less energy for rehabilitation: poor exercise tolerance
↑ Cholesterol	Key risk factor for CVD; evaluate other risk factors & assess risk for CAD prior to exercise
↑ Creatine	May have ↓ kidney function
↑ Creatine kinase	May have muscle injury, including heart; check isoenzymes (BB, MB, MM)
↑ Creatinine	May have ↓ kidney function

(Continued text on following page)

Rehabilitation Implications of General Chemistry (Continued)

Abnormal Lab Test Result	Implications for Rehabilitation
↓ Glucose	May be prediabetic or diabetic; check fasting glucose
↑ Iron	↑ O₂ carrying capacity; ↑ endurance/exercise tolerance
↓ LDH	Check isoenzyme for organ dysfunction; liver?
↓ Potassium	↑ risk of arrhythmia, myocardial muscle contractility heart?
↑ Potassium	↑ risk of arrhythmia
↑ Sodium	Affects resting threshold of action potentials; may have leg cramping
↑ T4 free	May have ↓ wt; will have difficulty w/wt loss until T4 NL
↓ Uric acid	May have painful foot joint(s)

Liver Function Tests	
Lab/Normal Values	**Meaning of Abnormal Results**
ALT/10-35 U/L	↑ Levels (10 × NL) w/acute hepatitis from acute infection & stay ↑ 1-3 mo ↓ in chronic hepatitis (4 × NL)
ALP/42-136 U/L	↑ Levels indicate bile duct blockage; if ALT & AST ↑, indicates ALP from liver; if ABN phosphorous & calcium, indicates ALP from bone
AST/0-35 U/L	↑ (10 × NL) w/acute hepatitis from acute viral infection, chronic hepatitis (4 × NL)
Bilirubin/ 0.3-1.0 mg/dL, Newborn 1-12 mg/dL, Critical: > 15 mg/dL	↓: Too many RBCs destroyed or liver not removing bilirubin; ↑ in infants: kills brain cells & causes mental retardation; may occur w/RH incompatibility; ↑ in adults: metabolic problems, bile duct obstruction, damage to liver or inherited abnormality

Liver Function Tests *(Continued)*

Lab/Normal Values	Meaning of Abnormal Results
Albumin/3.5-5 g/dL	↓ in liver & renal diseases, inflammation, shock & malnutrition; ↑ in dehydration
Total protein/7.0 g/dL	↓ in liver or kidney disorder or protein not being digested; ↓ albumin/globulin ratio in multiple myeloma or autoimmune diseases, cirrhosis or nephritic syndrome; ↑ in leukemia & genetic disorders

Emerging Risk Factors for CAD/Atherosclerosis

- Homocysteine
- C-reactive protein
- Lp(a)
- Thrombolytic factors (look at PT/PTT values)
- Endothelial dysfunction (↑ reactivity of arteries/arterioles: vasospasm or ↑ release of EDRF, resulting in ↑ LDL adhesion & atherosclerosis)
- Obesity
- Metabolic syndrome: three or more of the following:
  - Insulin resistance
    - Abnormal uric acid metabolism
    - Increased plasma uric acid concentration
    - Decreased renal clearance of uric acid
  - Elevated triglycerides
  - Hyperinsulinemia
  - Glucose intolerance
  - Decreased HDLs
  - Hypertension

Renal/Kidney Labs

Lab	NL Values	Rehabilitation Implications
BUN	8-25 mg/100 mL	↑ BUN in heart failure & renal failure; if ↑ creatinine, ↓ kidney functioning: indirect relationship between creatinine & GFR; ↑ creatinine means ↓ GFR
Creatinine	0.6-1.5 mg/100 mL	
Uric acid	3.0-7.0 mg/100 mL	

Cardiac Enzyme Markers

Lab/Normal Values	Elevation Timetable	Rehabilitation Implications
T 1/0.0-0.1 ng/mL T/< 0.18 ng/mL	↑ w/Any cardiac muscle damage; tested 2-3x w/acute chest pain; remains ↑ 1-2 wk after MI	Elevated markers indicate acute myocardial injury; pt should be evaluated & treated for myocardial injury prior to rehab interventions; see note below w/progression of values
CPK/40-150 U/L (F) 60-400 U/L (M)	Begins to rise 2-12 hr; returns to NL 2-4 days	
CPK-MB/<4%	Same as CK, also used to determine if clot-busting drugs working; will rise & fall faster w/drugs	
SGOT/AST/9-25 U/L (F); 10-40 U/L (M)	Begins to rise 6-24 hr; returns to NL 3-6 days	
LDH/70-180 U/L	Begins to rise 12-48 hr; returns to NL 7 days	
Myoglobin/10-95 ng/mL (M); 10-65 ng/mL (F)	Start to ↑ 2-3 hr after MI, peak 8-12 hr & returns to NL 24 hr after	
C-reactive protein/< 10 mg/L	↑ in acute inflammation	

Cardiac Enzyme Markers: Progression Over Time

Marker	Onset	Peak	Duration
Troponin – I	3-6 hr	12-24 hr	4-6 days
Troponin – T	3-5 hr	24 hr	10-15 days
CPK	4-6 hr	10-24 hr	3-4 days
CPK-MB*	4-6 hr	14-20 hr	2-3 days
SGOT/AST	12-18 hr	12-48 hr	3-4 days
LDH	3-6 days	3-6 days	6-7 days
Myoglobin	2-4 hr	6-10 hr	12-36 hr

*Rehab implications: elevated markers indicate acute injury to myocardium; PK-MB must peak & start to ↓ before pt begins OOB activities & rehabilitation

Lipids

	Normal Values	Deviations/Causes
Total cholesterol	<200 mg/dL Adults 125-200 mg/dL child	↑ Values ↑ risk for developing CAD; must look at total HDL ratio
HDL	Males >40 Females >50	↓ Values ↑ risk for developing CAD; must look at total HDL ratio
LDL	<100 mg/dL	↑ Values ↑ risk for developing CAD
VLDL	25-50%	↑ Values ↑ risk for CAD & diabetes
Triglycerides	<150 mg/dL	↑ Values may ↑ risk for CAD & diabetes
Total/HDL ratio	<4:1 ratio	↑ Ratio ↑ risk for CAD
Lp(a)	<10 mg/dL	↑ Indicates ↑ risk for thrombosis & CAD
HbA$_1$C	<6.5%	↑ % indicates blood glucose has been out of NL range within last 3 mo; indicates control of blood sugars for 3 mo

Other Cardiac Tests

	Normal Values	Deviations
Homocysteine	4-7 µmol/L	↓ Levels are a risk factor for CAD; ↓ in renal failure secondary to meds
C-reactive protein (1) High sensitivity CRP test for risk for CAD also called cardio CRP (2) Plain CRP test for inflammation or infection	<1.0 low CVD risk 1.0-3.0 average CVD risk 3.1-10 ↑ CVD risk	(1) ↓ Levels near 10 mg/L associated w/↑ risk of atherosclerosis (2) ↓ Levels near 100 mg/L in noncoronary inflammation, infection
BNP	< 100 pg/mL	↓ w/heart failure <500 goal for hospital discharge >700 decompensated heart failure
APC-R	< 2.0 (ratio)	↓ means ↑ for venous thromboembolic disease; CVD (women who smoke), & cerebrovascular disease; associated w/acute phase reactions
Verify now aspirin test (ARU) = aspirin reaction units	350-550 ARU = therapeutic range	> 550 nontherapeutic range/not reacting to aspirin

Hematology (CBC & Blood Counts)		
Lab Test	**NL Values**	**Deviations/Causes**
Blood volume	8/5-9.0% body wt (kg)	↓ Bleeding, burns, post surgery
RBC × 10^{12}/L	4.5–6.5 (M) 3.9-5.6 (F)	↑ Polycythemia vera, chronic lung disease, dehydration, congenital heart disease, CVD, high altitude exposure, smoking history, renal cell CA ↓ Anemias, renal failure (chronic), SLE, leukemia, bone marrow dysfunction, Hodgkin's disease, lymphomas, multiple myeloma, rheumatic fever
Hb (gm/dL)	13.5-17.5 (M) 11.5-15.5 (F)	↑ CHF, high altitude, dehydration, COPD ↓ Hemorrhage, anemia, cirrhosis, hemolysis
Hct (%)	40-52 (M) 36-48 (F)	Same as Hb
Leukocytes (WBC) (×10^9/L)	4-11	Same as differentials
Bands	0%-5%	↓ Immunosuppressive meds, aplastic anemia, radiation to bone marrow, lymphocytic & monocytic leukemia, agranulocytosis, antibiotics, viral infections
Basophils	0%-1%	↑ Myelofibrosis, polycythemia vera, Hodgkin's leukemia ↓ Anaphylactic reaction, stress, steroids, pregnancy, hyperthyroidism
		(Continued text on following page)

Hematology (CBC & Blood Counts) (Continued)

Lab Test	NL Values	Deviations/Causes
Eosinophils	1%-4%	↓ Allergies (asthma, hay fever), parasites (roundworm, fluke), malignancy, colitis ↑ Burns, SLE, acute infection, mononucleosis, CHF, infections w/neutrophilia +/or neutropenia, meds (ACTH), thyroxine, epinephrine
Lymphocytes	25%-40%	↓ Leukemia, viral infections diseases, viral infections w/exanthema (measles, rubella)
■ B-lymph	10%-20%	↓ in viral infection, leukemia, bone marrow cancer & radiation therapy. ↑ w/immune dyst (lupus & AIDS/HIV)
■ T-lymph	60%-80%	↓ in viral infection, leukemia, bone marrow cancer & radiation therapy. ↑ w/immune dyst (lupus & AIDS/HIV)
Monocytes	2%-8%	↓ in viral diseases, neoplasms, inflammatory bowel, collagen diseases, hematology disorders
Neutrophils	54%-75%	> bacterial infections, inflammatory diseases, carcinoma, trauma, stress, cortico-steroids, acute gout, diabetes, hemorrhage, hemolytic anemia < acute viral infections, bone marrow disease, nutritional deficiency (Vit B_{12}, folic acid)

Hematology (CBC & Blood Counts) *(Continued)*

Lab Test	NL Values	Deviations/Causes
Platelets (x 10^9/L)	150-450	↓ in bone marrow disease (leukemia/thrombocytopenia), long term bleeding problems, lupus, heparin or quinidine use, sulfa drugs, chemotherapy treatments ↑ in myeloproliferative disorders, living in high altitudes, strenuous exercise
ESR (mm/hr)	1-13 (M) 1-20 (F)	A nonspecific marker of inflammation ↑ (excessively ↑) indicates acute infection; mod ↑ w/inflammation, anemia, infection, pregnancy & ↑ age; ↑ in kidney failure, multiple myeloma, macroglobulinemia (tumors), & w/oral contraceptives, theophylline, penicillin, & dextran ↓ in polycythemia, leukocytosis, & some protein abnormalities; also ↓ w/aspirin, cortisone, & quinine

Rehab Implications

- ↓ RBC or ↓ Hb: less O_2 carrying capacity/↓ exercise tolerance/endurance
- ↑ WBC indicates infection: VS may be abnormally ↑
- ↓ platelets: ↑ risk of bleeding

Coagulation Studies

Lab/Normal Values	Deviations & Causes
ACT/175-225 sec	To monitor effect of high-dose heparin before, during, & after surgery ↓ = higher clotting inhibition (low platelets)
PTT or aPTT/ 20-35 sec Critical > 100	Used for unexplained bleeding ↓ w/clotting problems, ↑ when coag factor VIII elevated or acute tissue inflammation/trauma
Bleeding time/1-9 min (IVY)*	↓ w/defective platelet function, thrombocytopenia, von Willebrand's disease; also affected by drugs: dextran, indomethecin, & NSAIDS
Fibrinogen/150-400 mg/dL Critical < 100	↑ in acute infectious, coronary disease, stroke, MI, trauma, inflammatory disorders, breast/kidney/stomach cancer ↓ impairs ability to form clot, ↑ in liver disease, malnutrition, DIC, & cancers
INR/10-14 sec Critical >30	On anticoagulants: 2.0-3.0 for basic blood thinning, 2.5-3.5 for those w/higher clot risk (prosthetic heart valve, systemic emboli)
Plasminogen/80-92%	The inactive form of plasminogen participates in fibrinolysis; used to evaluate plasminogen of NL for plasma
Platelets/150 K-450 K/mm³↑	Critical levels < 50,000 or < 999,000 (thrombus) ↓ inflammatory disorders & myeloproliferative states, hemolytic anemias, cirrhosis, iron deficiency, acute blood loss ↑ in aplastic anemia, megaloblastic & iron deficiency anemias, uremia, DIC, etc.

Rehab Implications

*Caution w/↑ bleeding time, ↑ PTT or aPTT; ↓ platelets: should not be falling, bumping, or bruising w/activity.

†Critical level: platelets <50,000; may not be appropriate for rehab interventions

Urinalysis		
Lab	**NL Findings**	**Deviations & Causes**
Color/ appearance	Clear, yellow, straw	Lighter: urine diluted Dark: dehydration
Specific gravity	1.005-1.030	↓ means urine diluted; ↑ means urine concentrated
pH	4.6-8.0	↓ indicates acidosis, possibly secondary to ketones; ↑ indicates alkalosis
Glucose	Negative	Abnormal blood sugars
Leukocyte esterase	Negative	Positive indicates urinary tract infection
Nitrite	Negative	Positive: urinary tract infection
Ketones	Negative	Positive: blood sugars out of balance
Protein	2-8 mg/dL	↑ indicates ↓ renal function
Osmolality	300-900 mOsm/kg	Indicates diluted vs concentrated urine ↑ indicates dehydration, ↓ fluid overload
WBCs	3-4	↑ in urinary tract infection
RBCs	1-2	↑ w/damage to renal tubules
Crystals	Few/negative	↑ indicates presence of renal stones
RBC or WBC casts	Negative	↑ w/ upper urinary tract infections

CSF Analysis

Lab	NL Values
Pressure	50-180 mm H$_2$O
Appearance	Clear, colorless
Total protein	15-45 mg/dL
Prealbumin	2%-7%
Albumin	56%-76%
Alpha$_1$ globulin	2%-7%
Alpha$_2$ globulin	4%-12%
Beta globulin	8%-18%
Gamma globulin	3%-12%
Oligoclonal bands	None
IgG	<3.4 mg/dL
Glucose	500-800 mg/dL
Cell count	0-5 WBCs, NO RBCs
Chloride	118-132 mEq/L
Lactate dehydrogenase	10% of serum level
Lactic acid	10-20 mg/dL
Cytology	No malignant cells
Culture	No growth
Gram's stain*	Negative
India ink*	Negative
VDRL	Nonreactive

*Critical values: positive Gram's stain, India ink prep, or culture

Med Levels (Therapeutic Levels/Toxic Levels)

Med	Therapeutic	Toxic
Acetaminophen	5-20 mg/L	>25 mg/L
Amiodarone	0.5-2.0 mg/L	>2.5 mg/L
Carbamazepine	4.0-12.0 µg/mL	>12
Digoxin/Lanoxin*	0.5-2.0 µg/L	>2.2
Dilantin	10-20 µg/mL	>20
Lidocaine	1.5-5.0 mg/L	>7.0
Lithium	0.6-1.5 mEq/L	>1.5
Nitroprusside	<10 mg/dL	>10
Phenobarbital	15-40 µg/mL	>45
Procainamide	4-10 µg/mL	>15
Quinidine	1.2-4.0 µg/mL	>5.0
Salicylate	20-25 mg/100mL	>30
Theophylline**	10-20 µg/mL	>20

*Toxic levels Lanoxin: ↑ arrhythmias, changes on ECG, nausea

**↓Theophylline levels: therapeutic treatment not achieved for bronchodilation

Arterial Blood Gases

Lab	NL Range	Possible Causes of Deviations
pH	7.35-7.45	↑ **(Alkalosis)** Metabolic: ↑ Ca++, overdose of alkaline substance, vomiting Respiratory: hyperventilation, pulmonary embolus ↓ **(Acidosis)** Metabolic: diarrhea, renal failure, aspirin overdose Respiratory: hypoventilation, respiratory depression, CNS depression

(Continued text on following page)

Arterial Blood Gases (Continued)

Lab	NL Range	Possible Causes of Deviations
pO₂	75-100 mm Hg	↑ Values (hypoxia) in individuals w/lung disease, trauma, or infection; some interference w/O₂ getting into circulation; may require supplemental O₂
pCO₂	35-45 mm Hg	↑ Indicates hypercapnia/pt may be hyperventilating or blowing off too much CO₂ ↓ Indicates hypercapnia/pt retaining too much CO₂
HCO₃	22-26 mEq/L	↓ Levels indicate alkalosis: either a metabolic response to a respiratory acidosis or a primary metabolic disorder (e.g., vomiting, etc) ↑ Indicates acidosis: either metabolic response to respiratory alkalosis or a primary metabolic disorder (e.g., diabetic ketoacidosis, etc)
Base deficit/ excess	-2 - +2 mEq/L	Reflects concentration of bicarbonate in body; if > +3 or < -3 is critical
SpO₂	>95%	↑ Values indirectly indicate PO₂ in blood & O₂ dissociation; <90 % critical; may require supplemental O₂

Acid/Base Imbalances & Interpretation

	pH	pCO$_2$	HCO$_3$	Examples
Uncompensated respiratory acidosis	<7.35	>45	NL	Acute respiratory failure
Compensated respiratory acidosis	NL	>45	>26	Metabolically compensated respiratory failure
Uncompensated metabolic acidosis	<7.35	NL	<22	Diabetic ketoacidosis
Compensated metabolic acidosis	NL	<35	<22	
Acute respiratory alkalosis	>7.45	<35	NL	Hyperventilation ↑↑ pain
Compensated respiratory alkalosis	NL	<35	<22	
Uncompensated metabolic alkalosis	>7.45	NL	>26	Nausea, vomiting
Fully compensated metabolic alkalosis	NL	>45	>26	

MEDS

Traditional Medications

Type of Drug/Examples	
Anti-Alzheimer ■ Donepezil (Aricept) ■ Galantamine (Reminyl) ■ Rivastigmine (Exelon) ■ Tacrine (Cognex)	**Indication:** Management of dementia **Effect:** ↓ Amount of acetylcholine in CNS (inhibits cholinesterase); ↑ temperature ↑ cognitive function & LOC **Common side effects (most common):** Fatigue, dizziness, headache, diarrhea, nausea, incontinence, tremor, arthritis, muscle cramps **Precautions/Contraindications:** Contraind in hypersensitivity; cautious use w/hepatic reaction
Antianemics ■ Cyanocobalamin ■ Hydroxocobalamin (vit B₁₂ preparations) ■ Folic acid ■ Darbepoetin ■ Epoetin (Procrit) ■ Nandrolone (Decan) ■ Carbonyl iron (Feosol) ■ Ferrous fumarate ■ Ferrous gluconate ■ Ferrous sulfate ■ Iron (Dextran) (Slow Fe)	**Indication:** Prevention and treatment of anemias **Effect:** ↑ RBC and Hb production **Common side effects (most common):** 1. Oral Fe ↑ absorption of tetracyclines 2. Vit E ↓ response to Fe 3. Phenytoin (anticonvulsant) ↑ absorption of folic acid 4. Darbepoetin & epoetin may ↑ heparin need in hemodialysis Other side effects: Dizziness, headache, nausea, vomiting **Precautions/Contraindications:** Use parenteral iron cautiously in patients w/hypersensitive reactions or allergies; all are contraind in undiagnosed anemias, uncontrolled hypertension, hemolytic anemias

Traditional Medications *(Continued)*

Type of Drug/Examples	

Antianginals
Nitrates
■ Isosorbide dinitrate
■ Isordil
■ Nitroglycerin
Beta Blockers
■ Atenolol (Tenormin)
■ Carteolol (Cartrol)
	Indication: Nitrates
	Treat & prevent angina attacks &
	  acute angina
	**Ca+ Channel Blockers & Beta
	  Blockers**
	Effect: Nitrates
	Dilate coronary arteries; cause
	  systemic vasodilation
	Beta blockers
	↓ Myocardial O_2 consumption:
	  ↓ HR
	Ca+ Channel Blockers
	Common side effects (most com-
	mon): Hypotension/dizziness,
	particularly w/position changes.
	(orthostatic hypotension)
	Nitrates cause headaches; need
	to develop tolerance
	Precautions/Contraindications:
	  Beta blockers & Ca+ channel
	  blockers: contrain in
	  advanced heart block,
	  cardiogenic shock, and uncomp
	  heart failure

■ Labetalol (Normodyne)
■ Metoprolol (Toprol,
  Lopressor)
■ Nadolol (Corgard)
Ca+ Channel Blockers
■ Amlodipine (Norvasc)
■ Bepridil (Vascor)
■ Diltiazem (Cardizem)
■ Verapamil (Calan, Isoptin)
	Indication: Long-term mana-
	  gement of angina
	Effect: Smooth muscle arterial
	  relaxation (systemic)

(Continued text on following page)

MEDS

Traditional Medications (Continued)

Type of Drug/Examples	
Antianxiety **Benzodiazepines** ■ Alprazolam (Xanax) ■ Chlordiazepoxide (Librium) ■ Diazepam (Valium) ■ Lorazepam (Ativan) ■ Midazolam (Versed) ■ Oxazepam (Serax) **Others** ■ Buspirone (BuSpar) ■ Doxepin (Sinequan) ■ Hydroxyzine (Atarax/Vistaril) ■ Paroxetine (Paxil) ■ Prochlorperazine (Compazine) ■ Venlafaxine (Effexor)	**Indication:** Management of anxiety: general anxiety disorder; short-term: benzodiazepines; long term: buspirone, paroxetine, venlafaxine **Effect:** Generalized CNS depression; benzo-azepine: psychological or physical dependence **Common side effects (most common):** May cause daytime drowsiness; avoid driving & other activities requiring alertness Others: dizziness, lethargy, blurred vision, hypotension, physical dependence on meds **Precautions/Contraindications:** Avoid alcohol & other CNS depressants. Do not use if pregnant or breastfeeding. Not used in patients w/uncontrolled severe pain
Antiarrhythmics **Class IA** ■ Disopyramide (Norpace) ■ Moricizine (Ethmozine) ■ Procainamide (Procan) ■ Quinidine	**Indication:** Suppress cardiac arrhythmias Goal: ↑ symptoms & ↑ hemodynamic performance Classified by effect on cardiac conduct tissue **Effect: Class IA:** ↓ Na^{++} conduction, ↓ action potential & effective refraction period, ↑ membrane response **Common side effects (most common):** Dizziness, fatigue, headache, nausea, constipation, dry mouth, hypotension, ↑ arrhythmias, s/s of heart failure, hypoglycemia, fever **Precautions/Contraindications:** Take apical pulse before administering oral dose; (no <50 bpm); NOT used in individuals w/second- or third-degree heart block or in cardiogenic shock

Traditional Medications (Continued)

Type of Drug/Examples	
Class 1B ■ Lidocaine ■ Mexiletine (Mexitil) ■ Phenytoin (Dilantin) ■ Tocainide (Tonocard) **Class 1C** ■ Flecainide (Tambecor) ■ Propafenone (Rythmol) **Class II** ■ Acebutolol (Sectral) ■ Esmolol (Brevibloc) ■ Propranolol (Inderal) ■ Sotalol (Betapace) **Class III** ■ Amiodarone (Cordorone, Pacerone) ■ Dofetilide (Tikosyn) ■ Ibutilide (Corvert) **Class IV** ■ Diltiazem (Cardizem) ■ Verapamil **Others** ■ Adenosine ■ Atropine ■ Digoxin	**Effect: Class IB:** ↑ K+ conduction, ↓ action potential duration & refractory period **Class IC:** Slow conduction, ↓ phase 0 **Class II:** Interferes w/Na conduction, depresses cell membrane, ↓ automaticity, blocks ↑ symptom activity **Class III:** Interferes w/norepinephrine, ↑ AP & refractory period **Class IV:** ↑ AV nodal refractory period; calcium channel blocker
Antiasthmatics **Bronchodilators** ■ Albuterol (Proventil) ■ Epinephrine ■ Formoterol (Foradil) ■ Levalbuterol (Xopenex)	**Indication:** Management of acute & chronic episodes of reversible bronchoconstriction Goal: treat acute attacks & ↓ incidence & intensity of future attacks

(Continued text on following page)

Traditional Medications (Continued)

Type of Drug/Examples

Bronchodilators
- Metaproterenol (Alupent)
- Pirbuterol (Maxair)
- Salmeterol (Serevent)
- Terbutaline (Brethaire)
- Terbutaline

Corticosteroids
- Beclomethasone (Beclovent, Vanceril)
- Betamethasone
- Budesonide (Pulmicort)
- Cortisone
- Dexamethasone (Decadron)
- Flunisolide (Aerobid)
- Fluticasone (Flovent)
- Hydrocortisone
- Methylprednisolone
- Prednisone
- Triamcinolone (Azmacort)

Leukotriene Receptor Antagonist
- Zafirlukast (Accolate)

Mast Cell Stabilizers
- Cromolyn
- Nedocromil (Tilade)

Effect / Precautions

Effect: Bronchodilators & phosphodiesterase inhibitors ↑ intracellular cycles 3, 5 AMP by ↑ production or ↓ break down; corticosteroids ↑ airway inflammation; leukotriene receptor antagonists ↓ substances that induce bronchoconstriction

Common side effects (most common): Nervousness, restlessness, tremors, insomnias, palpitations, hyperglycemia, arrhythmias

Corticosteroids: depression, euphoria, personality changes, hypertension, peptic ulceration, ↑ wound healing, wt gain, cushingoid appearance

Precautions/Contraindications: Long-acting adrenergics, mast cell stabilizers, & inhaled corticosteroids: NOT used during acute attacks

Caution: adrenergics & anticholinergics w/CVD

Corticosteroids: NOT stopped abruptly; long-term use of systemic corticosteroids may ? bone & muscle mass & ↓ glycemic control

Traditional Medications *(Continued)*

Type of Drug/Examples	
Anticholinergics ■ Atropine ■ Benztropine ■ Biperidin ■ Glycopyrrolate ■ Ipratropium ■ Oxybutynin ■ Propantheline ■ Scopolamine ■ Tolterodine ■ Trihexyphenidyl	**Indication:** Brady arrhythmias, bronchospasm, nausea & vomiting from motion sickness, ↓ gastric secretory activity, used for Parkinson's disease **Effect:** Inhibit acetylcholine & inhibit action of acetylcholine at sites innervated by postganglionic cholinergic nerves **Common side effects** (most common): Drowsiness, dry mouth, dry eyes, blurred vision, constipation, inhibits absorption of other drugs: alters GI motility & transit time **Precautions/Contraindications:** Geriatric & pediatric pts more prone to adverse effects Use cautiously w/chronic renal, hepatic, pulmonary, or cardiac disease
Anticoagulants ■ Coumadin (Warfarin) ■ Fondaparinux ■ Dalteparin ■ Danaparoid ■ Enoxaparin ■ Tinzaparin ■ Argatroban ■ Bivalirudin ■ Lepirudin	**Indication:** Prevent & treat thromboembolic disorders: pulmonary emboli, atrial fibrillation, phlebitis Used for mgmt of MI **Effect:** Prevent clot formation & extension; heparin used first: rapid onset of action, followed by maintenance therapy **Common side effects** (most common): Dizziness, bleeding, anemia, thrombocytopenia **Precautions/Contraindications:** NOT indicated for coagulation disorders, ulcers, malignancies, recent surgery or active bleeding; use cautiously w/patients at risk for ↑ bleeding

(Continued text on following page)

Traditional Medications (Continued)

Type of Drug/Examples	
Anticonvulsants	**Indication:** ↑ Incidence & severity of seizures
Barbiturates	**Effect:** ↓ Abnormal neuronal dischar-ges in CNS; raise seizure threshold, alter levels of neurotransmitters, ↑ motor cortex or prevent spread of seizure activity
■ Pentobarbital	
■ Phenobarbital	
Benzodiazepines	
■ Diazepam	**Common side effects (most com-mon):** Ataxia, agitation, nystagmus, diplopia, hypertension, nausea, altered taste, anorexia, agranulocy-tosis, aplastic anemia, fever, rashes, hangover, nausea, hypotension
Other	
■ Acetazolamide	
■ Carbamazepine	
■ Divalproex sodium	
■ Gabapentin (Neurontin)	
■ Phenytoin (Dilantin)	**Precautions/Contraindications:** Cautious use w/severe hepatic or renal disease Caution w/pregnant females or breastfeeding mothers
■ Valproate sodium	
□ Zonisamide	
Antidepressants	**Indication: Depression**
MAO Inhibitors	Anxiety (doxepin), enuresis (impra-mine), chronic pain (amitriptyline, doxepin, imipramine, nortriptyline), smoking cessation (bupropion), Bulimia (fluoxetine), obsessive-compulsive disorder (fluoxetine, sertraline) & generalized anxiety (venlafaxine, paroxetine)
■ Phenelzine (Nardil)	
■ Tranylcypromine (Parnate)	
Serotonin Reup-take Inhibitors	
■ Citalopram (Celexa)	
■ Fluoxetine (Prozac)	
■ Fluvoxamine (Luvox)	**Effect:** Prevent reuptake of dopamine, norepinephrine, & serotonin by presynaptic neurons
■ Paroxetine	
■ Sertraline	
Tricyclics	**Result:** accumulation of neur-otransmitters
■ Amitriptyline	
■ Amoxapine	Most tricyclics: anticholinergic & sedative properties
■ Desipramine	

Traditional Medications *(Continued)*

Type of Drug/Examples	
■ Doxepin ■ Imipramine ■ Nortriptyline **Others** ■ Mirtazapine ■ Bupropion ■ Nefazodone ■ Trazodone ■ Venlafaxine	**Common side effects** (most common): Drowsiness, insomnia, dry eyes, dry mouth, blurred vision, constipation, orthostatic hypotension, dizziness **Precautions/Contraindications:** Hypersensitivity, glaucoma, pregnancy, lactation, immediate post MI, cautious w/geriatric pts w/preexisting CAD, prostate enlargement, slow titration
Antidiabetics ■ Acarbose ■ Glimepiride ■ Glipizide ■ Glyburide ■ Insulin ■ Metformin ■ Miglitol ■ Nateglinide ■ NPH insulin ■ Pioglitazone ■ Repaglinide ■ Rosiglitazone	**Indication:** Management of diabetes mellitus to control (lower) blood sugar **Effect:** Lower blood sugar **Common side effects** (most common): Hypoglycemia Dosage altered frequently due to stress, infection, exercise, changes in diet, etc. **Precautions/Contraindications:** Hypoglycemia, hypersensitivity, infection, stress or changes in diet may alter dosage Cautious in elderly patients
Antifungals ■ Amphotericin ■ Caspofungin ■ Fluconazole ■ Griseofulvin ■ Itraconazole ■ Ketoconazole ■ Terbinafine	**Indication:** Treatment of fungal infections **Effect:** Kill/stop growth of susceptible fungi: affects permeability of fungal cell membrane or protein synthesis **Common side effects** (most common): Skin irritation ↑ Risk of infection

(Continued text on following page)

Traditional Medications *(Continued)*	
Type of Drug/Examples	
	Precautions/Contraindications: May ↓ bone marrow function: use cautiously in pts w/↓ bone marrow function May also cause renal impairment
Antihistamines ■ Azatadine ■ Brompheniramine ■ Cetirizine (Zyrtec) ■ Chlorpheniramine (Chlor-Trimeton) ■ Cyproheptadine (Periactin) ■ Desloratidine ■ Hydroxyzine (Vistaril) ■ Loratadine (Claritan) ■ Promethazine (Phenergan)	**Indication:** Relief of allergy symptoms (rhinitis, urticaria, angioedema) Also used as adjunctive therapy in anaphylactic reactions **Effect:** Block effect of histamine at H1 receptor **Common side effects** (most common): Constipation, dry mouth, dry eyes, blurred vision, sedation **Precautions/Contraindications:** Contraind in hypersensitivity, narrow-angle glaucoma, prematurely born infants or newborns Cautious use w/elderly, pyloric obstruction, prostate hypertrophy, hyperthyroidism, cardiovascular, and liver disease
Antihypertensives: ACE Inhibitors ■ Benazepril ■ Captopril ■ Enlapril ■ Fosinopril	**Indication:** Treatment of ↑ BP & management of CHF/slows progression of L ventricle dysfunction Lisinopril: used in prevention of migraines

Traditional Medications (Continued)	
Type of Drug/Examples	
■ Lisinopril ■ Moexipril ■ Perindopril ■ Quinapril ■ Ramipril ■ Trandolapril	**Effect:** Lower BP, ↓ afterload in CHF, ↓ development of overt HF, ↑ survival after MI, blocks angiotensin I → vasoconstriction angiotension II Activates vasodilation bradykinins **Common side effects** (most common): Dizziness, fatigue, headache, rash, insomnia, angina, weakness, cough, hypotension, taste disturbance, cough, proteinuria, impotence, nausea, hyperkalemia, anorexia, diarrhea, neutropenia **Precautions/Contraindications:** Contraind in hypersensitivity, pregnancy, angioedema Cautious w/renal or hepatic impairment, hypovolemia Concurrent diuretic therapy, elderly, aortic stenosis, cerebrovascular or cardiac insufficiency, family hx of angioedema
Antihypertensives: Angiotension II Receptor Antagonists ■ Candesartan ■ Eprosartan ■ Irbesartan ■ Losartan ■ Telmisartan ■ Valsartan	**Indication:** Management of hypertension **Effect:** ↓ BP; blocks vasoconstriction effects of angiotension II at receptor sites: smooth muscle & adrenal glands **Common side effects** (most common): Dizziness, fatigue, headache, hypotension, diarrhea, drug-induced hepatitis, renal failure, hyperkalemia **Precautions/Contraindications:** Contraind in: hypersensitivity, pregnancy or lactation Cautious w/CHF, volume- or salt-depleted pts, pts w/diuretics, impaired renal, obstructive biliary disorders, age <18 yr

(Continued text on following page)

Traditional Medications (Continued)

Type of Drug/Examples	
Antihypertensives: **Beta blockers:** **Nonselective** ■ Carteolol ■ Carvedilol ■ Labetalol ■ Nadolol ■ Penbutolol ■ Pindolol ■ Propranolol ■ Timolol **Selective** ■ Acebutolol ■ Atenolol ■ Betaxolol ■ Bisoprolol ■ Metoprolol	**Indication:** Management of: hypertension & angina, may be used for prevention of MI **Effect:** Overall: ↑ HR & BP **Nonselective:** blocks stimulation of both beta-1 & beta-2 adrenergic recep sites **Selective:** blocks stimulation of beta-1 receptors; no effect on beta-2 receptors **Common side effects** (most common): Fatigue, weakness, impotence, anxiety, depression, mental status changes, memory loss, dizziness, drowsiness, insomnia, blurred vision, nervousness, nightmares, bradycardia, hypotension, CHF, bronchospasm (nonselective), vasoconstriction, hyper- & hypoglycemia, GI disturbance **Precautions/Contraindications:** Contraind: uncomp CHF, pulmonary edema, cardiogenic shock, bradycardia or heart block Cautious use w/renal or hepatic impairment, geriatric pts, pulmonary disease, diabetes, thyrotoxicosis, allergic reactions, & pregnancy
Antihypertensives: **Calcium Channel Blockers:**	**Indication:** Management of hypertension, angina pectoris, and vasospastic (Prinzmetal's angina)

Traditional Medications *(Continued)*

Type of Drug/Examples	
■ Amlodipine ■ Diltiazem ■ Felodipine ■ Isradipine ■ Nicardipine ■ Nifedipine ■ Nisoldipine ■ Verapamil	**Effect:** Systemic vasodilation: w/↓ BP, coronary vasodilation: ↓ frequency & attacks of angina. Inhibits transport of Ca++ → myocardial & vascular smooth muscle cells **Common side effects** (most common): Headache, peripheral edema, dizziness, fatigue, angina, bradycardia, hypotension, palpitations, flushing, nausea **Precautions/Contraindications:** Contraind in hypersensitivity & BP <90 mm Hg, bradycardia, second- or third-degree block or uncomp CHF **Cautious:** in severe hepatic impairment, geriatric pts, aortic stenosis, hx of CHF, pregnancy, lactation, or children
Antihypertensives Diuretics: ■ Chlorothiazide (diuril) ■ Chlorthalidone (hygroton) ■ Hydrochlorothiazide (hydrodiuril) ■ Indapamide ■ Metolazone	**Indication:** Management of hypertension or edema due to CHF or other causes; potassium-sparing diuretics have weak antihypertensive properties; used to conserve K+ **Effect:** ↑ Excretion of electrolytes and H₂O working on renal system **Common side effects** (most common): Hypokalemia, hyperuricemia, dizziness, lethargy, weakness, ↓ BP,

(Continued text on following page)

Traditional Medications (Continued)

Type of Drug/Examples	
Aminoglycosides: ■ Gentamicin ■ Kanamycin ■ Neomycin ■ Streptomycin ■ Tobramycin **Cephalosporins** ■ Cefadroxil (Duricef) ■ Cefazolin (Ancef) ■ Ceftriaxone (Ceftin) ■ Cephalexin (Keflex)	**Indication:** Treat/prevent bacterial infections **Effect:** Kill/inhibit growth of pathogenic bacteria; do not work against fungi or viruses **Common side effects** (most common): Diarrhea, nausea, vomiting, rashes, urticaria, seizures, dizziness, drowsiness, headache **Precautions/Contraindications:** Contraind w/hypersensitivity to specific drugs
Antihypertensives: **Others:** ■ Clonidine ■ Doxazosin ■ Fenoldopam ■ Guanabenz ■ Guanadrel ■ Guanfacine ■ Methyldopa ■ Minoxidil ■ Nitroprusside ■ Prazosin □ Terazosin	**Indication:** Treatment of essential hypertension; therapy initiated w/agents w/minimum side effects, w/more potent drugs added to control BP **Effect:** To ↓ diastolic BP to <90 mm Hg to lowest tolerated level Antiadrenergic properties (peripheral & central) & vasodilation **Common side effects** (most common): Dizziness, hypotension, weakness, dry mouth, bradycardia, sodium retention, GI problems **Precautions/Contraindications:** Cautious w/renal dysfunction & uncompensated CHF
	anorexia, cramping, hyperglycemia, dehydration, hyponatremia, muscle cramps, pancreatitis **Precautions/Contraindications:** Contraind in hypersensitivity; cautious use w/renal or hepatic disease

Traditional Medications *(Continued)*

Type of Drug/Examples	
Fluoroquinolones ■ Ciprofloxacin (Cipro) ■ Enoxacin (Penetrex) ■ Gatifloxacin (Tequin) ■ Levofloxacin (Levaquin) **Macrolides** ■ Azithromycin (Zithromax) ■ Clarithromycin (Biaxin) ■ Erythromycin **Penicillins** ■ Amoxicillin (Amoxil) ■ Ampicillin **Sulfonamides** ■ Sulfacetamide ■ Sulfamethoxazole **Tetracyclines** ■ Doxycycline ■ Minocycline ■ Tetracycline **Others** ■ Cloxacillin (Cloxapen) ■ Dicloxacillin (Dycill) ■ Nafcillin (Nallpen) ■ Vancomycin	Cautious use w/pregnant or lactating women, hepatic or renal insufficiency Prolonged use of broad-spectrum drugs may lead to additional infection w/fungi or resistant bacteria
Antineoplasms **Alkylating Agents** ■ Busulfan ■ Chlorambucil ■ Melphalan ■ Procarbazine **Anthracyclines** ■ Doxorubicin ■ Epirubicin	**Indication:** Treatment of solid tumors, lymphomas, & leukemias; often combine meds **Effect:** Various agents have various effects; may affect DNA synthesis or function, alter immune function or hormonal status; may affect other cells besides neoplastic cells

(Continued text on following page)

Traditional Medications (Continued)

Type of Drug/Examples	
Antitumor Antibiotic ■ Bleomycin ■ Mitomycin	**Common side effects** (most common): Nausea, vomiting, alopecia, anemia, leukopenia, thrombocytopenia, GI disturbances, pulmonary fibrosis, itching, rashes, arthralgia, myalgia, chills, fever, infection, hot flashes **Precautions/Contraindications:** Contraind in previous bone marrow depression or hypersensitivity, pregnancy, or lactation Use w/caution in pts w/active infections, ↑ bone marrow reserve, radiation therapy, or debilitating illness
Hormonal Agents ■ Estramustine ■ Letrozole ■ Tamoxifen **Vinca Alkaloids** ■ Vinblastine ■ Vincristine	
Antiparkinson Agents ■ Benztropine ■ Biperiden ■ Bromocriptine ■ Carbidopa ■ Entacapone ■ Levodopa ■ Pergolide ■ Pramipexole ■ Ropinirole ■ Selegiline	**Indication:** Treatment of Parkinson's disease of various causes: degenerative, toxic, infective, neoplastic, or drug-induced **Effect:** Reduction of rigidity and tremors; restores balance of major neurotransmitters: acetylcholine & dopamine; ↓ dopamine results in ↑↑ cholinergic activity **Common side effects** (most common): Blurred vision, dry eyes, dry mouth, constipation, confusion, depression, dizziness, headache, sedation, weakness **Precautions/Contraindications:** Contraind in pts w/narrow-angle glaucoma Use cautiously w/severe cardiac disease, pyloric obstruction, or prostate enlargements

Traditional Medications *(Continued)*

Type of Drug/Examples	
Antiplatelets ■ Aspirin ■ Cilostazol ■ Clopidogrel (Plavix) ■ Dipyridamole (Persantine) ■ Epifibatide (Integrilin) ■ Ticlopidine (Ticlid) ■ Tirofiban (Aggrastat)	**Indication**: Treatment and prevention of thromboembolic events (stroke, MI) Dipyridamole used after cardiac surgery **Effect**: Inhibit platelet aggregation Some inhibit phosphordiesterase **Common side effects** (most common): Headache, dizziness, hypotension, palpitations, tachycardia, nausea, diarrhea, gastritis, GI bleeding **Precautions/Contraindications**: Contraind in hypersensitivity, ulcer disease, active bleeding, recent surgery Use w/caution in pts at risk for bleeding (surgery or trauma), hx of GI bleeding or ulcers
Antipsychotics ■ Chlorpromazine ■ Clozapine ■ Fluphenazine ■ Haloperidol (Haldol) ■ Olanzapine (Zyprexa) ■ Prochlorperazine (Compazine) ■ Quetiapine (Seroquel) ■ Risperidone ■ Thioridazine (Mellaril) ■ Trifluoperazine ■ Ziprasidone (Geodon)	**Indication**: Treatment of psychoses: acute and chronic; treatment of psychomotor activity associated w/psychoses **Effect**: Decrease s/s of psychoses; block dopamine receptors in brain; alter dopamine release and turnover Anticholinergic effects peripherally **Common side effects** (most common): Extrapyramidal reactions, dyskinesia, sedation, photosensitivity, blurred vision, dry eyes, dry mouth, leukopenia, constipation, hypotension

(Continued text on following page)

Traditional Medications (Continued)

Type of Drug/Examples	
	Precautions/Contraindications: Contraind in hypersensitivity, w/narrow angle glaucoma, & w/CNS depression Cautions w/CAD; severely ill, debilitated pts, diabetics, w/respiratory insufficiency, hypertrophy of prostate, intestinal obstruction
Antirheumatics **Corticosteroids** ■ Betamethasone ■ Cortisone ■ Dexamethasone ■ Hydrocortisone ■ Methylprednisolone ■ Prednisone **Disease-Modifying Antirheumatics** ■ Azathioprine (Imuran) ■ Etanercept (Enbrel) ■ Hydroxychloroquine ■ Infliximab ■ Leflunomide ■ Methotrexate ■ Penicillamine **NSAIDs** ■ See below	**Antirheumatics** **Indication:** Management of pain & swelling in RA, ↑ progression of disease, & joint destruction; preserve joint function **Effect:** NSAIDs & corticosteroids are anti-inflammatory meds; DMARDs suppress autoimmune response (cell-mediated immunity & altered antibody formation) **Common side effects** (most common): Steroids: depression, nausea, euphoria, anorexia, hypertension, muscle wasting, osteoporosis, cushingoid appearance, ↑ wound healing, adrenal suppression, personality changes, fluid retention NSAIDs: dizziness, drowsiness, nausea, constipation, rashes, palpitations, ↓ bleeding time DMARDs: anemia, leukopenia, anorexia, nausea, chills, fever, rash, retinopathy, Raynaud's phenomenon **Precautions/Contraindications:** Contraind in hypersensitivity NO NSAIDs if allergic to aspirin Steroids: NOT w/active untreated infections Caution w/hx of GI bleeding, diabetics DMARDs: NOT used in active infections, underlying malignancy, & uncontrolled diabetes

Traditional Medications *(Continued)*

Type of Drug/Examples	
Antiulcer **Antacids** ■ Aluminum hydroxide ■ Magaldrate **Antiinfectives** ■ Amoxicillin ■ Clarithromycin **Histamine H$_2$-Receptor** ■ Antagonists ■ Cimetidine (Tagamet) ■ Famotidine (Pepcid) ■ Nizatidine (Axid) ■ Ranitidine (Tritec) **Other** ■ Esomeprazole (Nexium) ■ Lansoprazole (Prevacid) ■ Bismuth subsalicylate	**Indication:** Treat & prevent peptic ulcer or gastroesophageal reflux disease **Effect:** Antiinfective act on *Helicobacter pylori*, antacids neutralize stomach acid/protect ulcer surface from further damage **Common side effects** (most common): May interfere w/absorption of other oral meds, confusion, dizziness, drowsiness, ↓ sperm count, impotence, altered taste, black tongue **Precautions/Contraindications:** Hypersensitivity Cautious w/renal impairment & elderly
Antiviral ■ Acyclovir ■ Amantadine ■ Cidofovir ■ Dososanol ■ Famciclovir ■ Foscarnet ■ Ganciclovir ■ Oseltamivir ■ Penciclovir ■ Ribavarin ■ Valacyclovir ■ Valganciclovir ■ Vidarabine ■ Zanamivir	**Indication:** Management of viruses: acyclovir: herpes virus & chickenpox; oseltamivir & zanamivir: influenza A; cidofovir, ganciclovir, valganciclovir, foscarnet: CMV; vidarabine: ophthalmic viruses **Effect:** Inhibit viral replication **Common side effects** (most common): Acyclovir may cause CNS toxicity; foscarnet ↑ risk of seizures Other side effects: Dizziness, headache, nausea, diarrhea, vomiting, trembling, pain, phlebitis, joint pain

(Continued text on following page)

Traditional Medications *(Continued)*	
Type of Drug/Examples	
	Precautions/Contraindications: Contraind w/previous hypersensitivity Cautious w/renal impairment (dosage must be adjusted)
Bone Resorption Inhibitors ■ Alendronate (Fosamax) ■ Etidronate (Didronel) ■ Pamidronate (Aredia) ■ Raloxifene (Evista)	**Indication:** Treatment & prevention of osteoporosis **Effect:** Inhibit bone resorption/ inhibit osteoclast activity Bind to estrogen receptors **Common side effects** (most common): Abdominal pain, distention, constipation, diarrhea, musculoskeletal pain **Precautions/Contraindications:** Contraind: hypersensitivity, hypocalcemia, or women w/hx of thromboembolic disease Cautious w/renal impairment
CNS Stimulants ■ Amphetamine ■ Dexmethylphenidate ■ Dextroamphetamine ■ Methylphenidate (Ritalin) ■ Pemoline	**Indication:** Treatment of narcolepsy & management of ADHD **Effect:** ↑ levels of neurotransmitters in CNS, stimulation of respiratory and CNS, ↑ motor activity & mental alertness, ↓ sense of fatigue **Common side effects** (most common): Hyperactivity, insomnia, tremor, hypertension, palpitations, tachy, anorexia, constipation, dry mouth, rashes, hypersensitivity reactions

Traditional Medications *(Continued)*	
Type of Drug/Examples	
	Precautions/Contraindications: Contraind: hypersensitivity, pregnant & lactating women, hyperexcitable states Cautious: w/psychotic personalities or suicidal/homicidal, pts w/hx of CAD; diabetes; and elderly
Lipid Lowering ■ Atorvastatin (Lipitor) ■ Cholestyramine (Questran) ■ Colesevelam (Welchol) ■ Colestipol (Colestid) ■ Crestor ■ Fenofibrate (Tricor) ■ Fluvastatin (Lescol) ■ Gemfibrozil (Lopid) ■ Lovastatin (Mevacor) ■ Niacin ■ Pravastatin (Pravachol) ■ Simvastatin (Zocor) ■ Vytorin	**Indication:** To ↓ blood lipids/↓ risk of morbidity & mortality of atherosclerotic CVD **Effect:** Inhibit enzymes in cholesterol synthesis or bind cholesterol in GI tract **Common side effects** (most common): Abdominal discomfort, constipation, nausea, rashes MUSCLE PAIN/ACHING not associated w/exercise; may be sign of toxicity to drug **Precautions/Contraindications:** Hypersensitivity, complete biliary obstruction Cautious: w/hx of constipation, liver disease
NSAIDs ■ Aspirin ■ Celecoxib ■ Choline salicylate ■ Flurbiprofen ■ Ibuprofen ■ Indomethacin ■ Ketoprofen	**Indication:** Control of mild → mod pain, fever & inflammatory conditions: osteo- & rheumatoid arthritis **Effect:** Analgesia, anti-inflammatory, and ↓ fever; inhibits synthesis of prostaglandins

(Continued text on following page)

Traditional Medications (Continued)

Type of Drug/Examples	
■ Nabumetone ■ Naproxen ■ Oxaprozin ■ Piroxicam ■ Proxicam ■ Salsalate ■ Sulindac ■ Tolmetin ■ Valdecoxib	**Common side effects** (most common): Dizziness, drowsiness, nausea, constipation, palpitations, rashes, prolonged bleeding time **Precautions/Contraindications:** if allergic to aspirin: NO NSAIDs Cautious: w/hx of bleeding disorders, including GI Cautious use w/hepatic, renal & cardiovascular disease
Skeletal Muscle Relaxants ■ Baclofen ■ Carisoprodol ■ Chlorzoxazone ■ Cyclobenzaprine ■ Dantrolene ■ Diazepam ■ Metaxalone ■ Methocarbamol ■ Orphenadrine	**Indication:** Management of & relief of pain in acute musculoskeletal conditions **Effect:** Centrally acting (all except dantrolene) Inhibit reflexes at spinal level & may affect bowel & bladder function **Common side effects** (most common): Nausea, dizziness, drowsiness, fatigue, weakness, constipation, hyperglycemia May cause muscle weakness **Precautions/Contraindications:** Contraind in pts who use spasticity for functional activities including posture & balance Cautious w/previous liver disease

The Components of Patient/Client Management

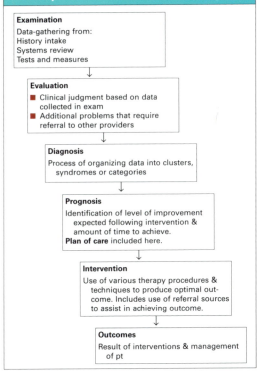

Examination

Data-gathering from:
History intake
Systems review
Tests and measures

Evaluation

■ Clinical judgment based on data collected in exam
■ Additional problems that require referral to other providers

Diagnosis

Process of organizing data into clusters, syndromes or categories

Prognosis

Identification of level of improvement expected following intervention & amount of time to achieve.
Plan of care included here.

Intervention

Use of various therapy procedures & techniques to produce optimal outcome. Includes use of referral sources to assist in achieving outcome.

Outcomes

Result of interventions & management of pt

Clinical Problem-Solving

- [ ] 1. Identify patient's symptoms
- [ ] 2. Determine symptoms to be assessed
- [ ] 3. Identify characteristics of relevant symptoms
- [ ] 4. Develop priority list of problems to be assessed
- [ ] 5. Identify procedures to examine the symptoms
- [ ] 6. Perform the examination
- [ ] 7. Interpret the results of the examination (evaluation)
- [ ] 8. Establish diagnosis
- [ ] 9. Identify goals & plan of treatment
- [ ] 10. Provide interventions
- [ ] 11. Evaluate effect of interventions
- [ ] 12. Modify treatment program as indicated

Documentation

General Principles of "Best Practice" Documentation

Principles	Documentation Details
Consistent w/payer rules & regulations	**Medicare:** Know local coverage determination (LCD or LMRP) Know **terminology** used: ■ Medically necessary ■ Skilled ■ Qualified provider ■ Supervision ■ Practice setting **Commercial payers:** Review coverage: contact specific payers for details

General Principles of "Best Practice" Documentation* *(Cont'd)*

Principles	Documentation Details
Provides necessary detail pertaining to pt's condition	Answer question: "Why does pt need these services?" Physician referral w/diagnosis Rehab exam including: ■ Subjective info: symptoms, impact on daily life & function ■ Objective info: impairments, functional limitations and disability
Includes health-care provider's assessment of need for rehab service	■ Answer question: "How will pt benefit from service & how will service be administered?" ■ Define "needs" for skilled services ■ Identify measurable goals w/time frames, functional in nature & based on objective data
Outlines a detailed plan of care specific for individual pt	■ Specific modality/exercises w/frequency, duration, & extent of monitoring or supervision ■ Individualized
Provides detail of interventions delivered	Includes specific interventions, responses to interventions, & progress toward goals Services provided billed appropriately
Describes a prognosis, with a time frame & expected outcomes	Relate to PT diagnosis & reflect need for skilled care

*Web sites/References: cms.hhs.gov/mcd/search.asp;aacvpr.org; specific payers' Web sites; *Guide to PT Practice*; ICD-9 code book; AMA CPT guide.

SOAP NOTE Format

Component	Specific Details Included in Component
Subjective	Problem: chief complaint Information reported by pt related to management: ■ Pain or pain behavior ■ Current medications ■ Home situation ■ Past medical history ■ Prior level of functioning ■ Patient's goals ■ Current level of function
Objective	Past medical hx from medical record Results of objective measurements/observations Description of any treatment provided Description of patient education provided Documentation of communication w/any other referrals/disciplines/MD
Assessment	Assessment of pt's problems for other health professionals to understand, overview of problems, & need for skilled intervention, to include: ■ Problem list ■ Goals: long-term (end of therapy) and short-term (interim goals) ■ Measurable, realistic, observable, time span, functional ■ Summary: PT impression including diagnosis & prognosis (guidance terminology)
Plan	■ Frequency per day/week ■ Treatment to be given ■ Education ■ Equipment needs ■ Plans for further assessment/referral ■ Criteria for discharge

Outcome Tools

Functional Assessment Outcome Tools

Test	Description
Barthel Index	Measures functional independence in ADLs
Borg Rating of Perceived Exertion	Perceived effort w/activity (6-20 scale or 0-10 scale)
Box and Block Test	Gross dexterity w/grasp & release/unilateral assessment
Canadian Occupational Performance Measure	Pt's assessment of performance in self-care over time
Clinical Outcome Variable Scale	Assessment of physical mobility
Disabilities of the arm, shoulder, & hand	UE disability quantified: physical, social, & symptom measures
Functional Assessment System of Lower Extremity Dysfunction	LE function in arthritic patients (20 variables, 5-point scale)
Functional Independence Measure	Functional independence assessed in 23 items
Katz ADL index	Degree of Dependence (8-point scale): mostly in elderly, also used in children
Kenny Self-Care Evaluation	Assessment of ADLs
Klein-Bell ADL Scale	Assessment of ADL of adults w/disability (170 items)
Level of Rehabilitation Scale	Assessment of independence in ADLs, mobility, and communication
Lower Extremity Activity Profile	LE function (self-care and mobility: 23 items)

(Continued text on following page)

Functional Assessment Outcome Tools (Continued)

Test	Description
Visual Analogue Scale for Dyspnea	Pt's perceptions of dyspnea; used with activities
Upper Extremity Functional Scale	UE function in the workplace
Timed "Up and Go" Test	Mobility of frail elderly; timed rise from chair, walk for 3 M, return to sit
Timed Stands Test	Lower extremity strength in pts w/arthritis
Timed Walk Tests (3-, 6-, 12-min)	Functional performance during ambulation; originally tested in chronic lung disease patients
Self-Paced Walking Test	Estimate max O₂ uptake following walk of 128 M at 3 paces
Seattle Angina Questionnaire	Assess function in pts w/angina symptoms
Rivermead Mobility Index	Mobility in pts w/neurological conditions
PULSES Profile	Function in chronically ill institutionalized persons
Patient Evaluation Conference System	Changes in function in pts in rehabilitation (79 items)
Older Americans Resources & Services Scale–Instrumental Activities of Daily Living	Functional ability & needs for home services in older adults
Lower Extremity Functional Scale	LE function in pts w/musculoskeletal disorders (20 items)

Health Status/Quality of Life Outcome Tools

Test	Description
Arthritis Impact Measurement Scales	Quantifies health status of RA over physical, social, and mental domains
Chronic Respiratory Disease Questionnaire	QOL in pts w/chronic lung disease
EuroQoL-5D (European Quality of Life Scale)	Health-care QOL
Health Utilities Index	Health-related QOL
Living with Heart Failure Questionnaire	QOL in pts/w congestive heart failure
Nottingham Health Profile	Health status w/musculoskeletal disorders (38 items)
St. George's Respiratory Questionnaire	Health-related QOL in pts w/chronic lung disease
Short Form Health Survey (SF-36)	Perceived health status; nondisease-specific (36 items)
12-Item Short Form Health Survey	Shorter version of SF-36
Sickness Inventory Profile	Perceived health status in nondisease-specific populations

Musculoskeletal-Specific Outcome Tools

Spine/low back-specific outcome tool	Dual inclinometer method of measuring spinal mobility	Spinal mobility
	Inclinometer method (single) of measuring spinal mobility	Spinal mobility
	Modified Schober method for measuring spinal mobility	Spinal mobility

(Continued text on following page)

Health Status/Quality of Life Outcome Tools *(Continued)*		
	Numeric Pain Rating Scale	Pain intensity in pts w/ muscular disorders
	Oswestry Low Back Pain Disability Questionnaire	Perceived disability due to low back pain
	Roland & Morris Disability Questionnaire	Disability index for patients w/low back pain
	Sorensen Test for Endurance of Back Muscles	Back muscle function (in prone position)
	Visual Analogue Scale for Pain	Pt's perceptions of pain; used w/activities
UE-specific	Box and Block Test	Gross dexterity w/grasp & release/unilateral assessment
	Disabilities of the arm, shoulder, & hand	UE disability quantified: physical, social, & symptom measures
	Upper Extremity Functional Scale	UE function in the workplace
	Wolf Motor Function Test	Assesses speed of movement in 15 UE movements post traumatic brain injury & CVA
LE-specific	Functional Assessment System of Lower Extremity Dysfunction	LE function in arthritic patients (20 variables, 5-point scale)
	Lower Extremity Activity Profile	LE function (self-care & mobility: 23 items)
	Lower Extremity Functional Scale	LE function in pts w/ muscular disorders (20 items)
	Timed Stands Test	LE strength in pts w/ arthritis

👶 Pediatric-Specific Outcome Tools

Alberta Infant Motor Scale	Assesses delays in development of motor performance: 58 items
Bayley Scales of Infant Development	Functional development from 1–42 mo
Bruininks-Oseretsky Test of Motor Proficiency	Developmental motor functioning for ages 4.5–14.5 yr (46 items)
Gross Motor Function Measure	Gross motor function in children w/cerebral palsy & Down syndrome compared with 5-yr-old child
Gross Motor Performance Measure	Quality of movement in children w/cerebral palsy (20 items)
Peabody Developmental Motor Scale, 2nd ed	Gross and fine motor skills in children from birth to 6 yr
Pediatric Evaluation of Disability Inventory	Mobility, self-care, & social function 6 mo–7 yr
WeeFIM (Functional Independence for Children)	Change in disability in children over time

Stroke-Specific Outcome Tools

Test	Items Examined
Action Research Arm Test	UE function after a stroke: 4 subscales
Canadian Neurological Scale	Post acute CVA neuro-status: mental status, motor function, & response
Chedoke-McMaster Stroke Assessment	Impairments & disability post CVA
Emory Functional Ambulation Profile	Assessment of ambulation capability post CVA
Frenchay Arm Test	Arm function recovery post CVA

(Continued text on following page)

Stroke-Specific Outcome Tools (Continued)

Test	Items Examined
Fugl-Meyer Assessment of Sensorimotor Recovery after Stroke	Recovery post CVA
Motor Assessment Scale	Motor recovery post CVA
Stroke-Adapted Sickness Impact Profile	QOL post CVA
Stroke Impact Scale	Functional assessment post CVA
Wolf Motor Function Test	Assesses speed of movement in 15 UE movements post traumatic brain injury & CVA

Other Outcome Tools

	Test	Items Examined
Balance	Activity-Specific Balance Confidence Scale	Determine confidence in not losing balance: 16-item scale
	Berg Balance Scale	Balance/maintenance of posture w/14 challenges
	Functional Reach Test	Balance
Depression	Beck Depression Inventory	Depression symptoms and function
Diet assessment	Diet Habit Survey	Saturated fat, salt, & complex carbohydrate intake
	MEDFICTS (meat, eggs, dairy, fried foods, baked goods, convenience foods, table fats, snacks)	Dietary fat intake
Pain assessment	Numeric Pain Rating Scale	Pain intensity in pts w/musculoskeletal disorders
	Visual Analogue Scale for Pain	Pt's perceptions of pain; used w/activities

Modified from Rothstein, Roy, & Wolf: The Rehabilitation Specialist's Handbook, Table 8-3, FA Davis, 2005.

Reimbursement Coding

Therapists often use the following CPT codes for charging for their services. Providers of rehab therapy services must refer to their Local Review Medicare Policy and their specific insurance carriers regarding payment for their services in using these codes as well as whether these codes can be used for the specific ICD-9 diagnostic code(s) that are assigned to each patient when referred to therapy. See AMA *Guide to CPT Coding* for specific information on CPT coding and descriptions.

To identify LMRPs for therapy services:
cms.hhs.gov/mcd/search.asp

More common CPT codes used in therapy: (* are timed codes)

97001:	Physical Therapy Evaluation
97002:	Physical Therapy Re-evaluation
97005:	Occupational Therapy Evaluation
97010:	Hot or cold packs
97012:	Traction, mechanical
97014:	Electrical stimulation (unattended)
97016:	Vasopneumatic services
97018:	Paraffin bath
97020:	Microwave
97022:	Whirlpool
97024:	Diathermy
97026:	Infrared
97028:	Ultraviolet
97032*:	Electrical stimulation (manual), 15 minutes
97033*:	Iontophoresis,
97034*:	Contrast baths, 15 minutes
97035*:	Ultrasound, 15 minutes
97036*:	Hubbard tank, 15 minutes
97039:	Unlisted modality
97110*:	Therapeutic exercise, 15 minutes
97112*:	Neuromuscular reeducation, 15 minutes
97113*:	Aquatic therapy with therapeutic exercise, 15 minutes
97116*:	Gait training, 15 minutes
97124*:	Massage, 15 minutes
97139:	Unlisted physical medicine procedure
97140*:	Manual therapy techniques, 15 minutes
97150:	Therapeutic procedures, group

(Continued text on following page)

Reimbursement Coding (Continued)

97504*:	Orthotics fitting and training, 15 minutes
97520*:	Prosthetics training, 15 minutes
97530*:	Therapeutic activities, 15 minutes
97532*:	Development of cognitive skills, one-on one, each 15 minutes
97533*:	Sensory integrative techniques, one-on-one, each 15 min
97535*:	Self care and home management, 15 min
97537*:	Community/work reintegration, 15 min
97542*:	Wheelchair management/propulsion training, 15 min
97545:	Work hardening/conditioning, initial 2 hours
97546:	Work hardening/conditioning, each additional hour
97597:	Removal of devitalized tissue from wound, selective debridement w/o anesthesia, less than or equal to 20 sq. cms
97598:	Debridement of total wound surface area of >20 sq. cm
97602:	Non-selective debridement
97605:	Negative pressure wound therapy; total wound surface area < or equal to 50 sq. cm
97606:	Negative pressure wound therapy, total wound surface area: 50 sq. cm
97703*:	Checkout for orthotic/prosthetic use, estab patient, each 15 min
97750*:	Physical performance test or measurement, each 15 min (Report required to accompany claim)
97755:	Assistive technology assessment

Time Increments for Billing Purposes

Time (min)	0–<8	>7–<23	>22–<38	>37–<53	>52–<68
Billable time (units)	0	1	2	3	4

Modifiers used

-22:	Unusual procedural services
-52:	Reduced services
-59:	Distinct procedural service
-76:	Repeat procedure by same physician
-32:	Mandated services (e.g., workers compensation requires functional capacity evaluation)
-99:	Multiple modifiers

Index (cont. on back cover)

ISBN 10: 0-8036-1398-9

ISBN 13: 978-0-8036-1398-0